How Ethical Systems Change:
Eugenics, the Final Solution, Bioethics

Sheldon Ekland-Olson and Julie Beick

Mandatory sterilization laws enacted in dozens of states coast-to-coast and approved by the U.S. Supreme Court formed the initial pillar for what became the Final Solution. Following World War II, there was renewed interest in a more inclusive view of social worth and the autonomy of the individual. Social movements were launched to secure broad-based revisions in civil and human rights. This book is based on a hugely popular undergraduate course taught at The University of Texas, and is ideal for those interested in science-based policy, the social construction of social worth, social problems, and social movements.

Sheldon Ekland-Olson joined The University of Texas at Austin after completing his graduate work at the University of Washington in Seattle and Yale Law School. He is currently the Bernard and Audre Rapoport Centennial Professor of Liberal Arts. He served for five years as Dean of the College of Liberal Arts and then for eight years as Executive Vice President and Provost of the university. He has authored or co-authored several books and numerous articles on criminal justice, prison reform, and capital punishment. Widely recognized for his commitment to teaching undergraduates, he is the recipient of numerous teaching awards. His current interests are reflected in the book *Who Lives, Who Dies, Who Decides?* (Routledge, 2012).

Julie Beicken is a doctoral student in the Department of Sociology at The University of Texas at Austin. Her research interests include political sociology, social movements, eugenics, the Supreme Court, and reproductive technologies. Julie received her Master's degree in 2009 for her thesis "Eugenics: An Elite Social Movement." She has published book reviews in *Women's Studies International Forum* and *Critical Mass*.

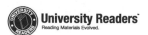 THE SOCIAL ISSUES COLLECTION™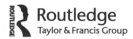

Framing 21st Century Social Issues

The goal of this new, unique Series is to offer readable, teachable "thinking frames" on today's social problems and social issues by leading scholars. These are available for view on http://routledge.customgateway.com/routledge-social-issues.html.

For instructors teaching a wide range of courses in the social sciences, the Routledge *Social Issues Collection* now offers the best of both worlds: originally written short texts that provide "overviews" to important social issues *as well as* teachable excerpts from larger works previously published by Routledge and other presses.

As an instructor, click to the website to view the library and decide how to build your custom anthology and which thinking frames to assign. Students can choose to receive the assigned materials in print and/or electronic formats at an affordable price.

Available

Body Problems
Running and Living Long in a Fast-Food Society
Ben Agger

Sex, Drugs, and Death
Addressing Youth Problems in American Society
Tammy Anderson

The Stupidity Epidemic
Worrying About Students, Schools, and America's Future
Joel Best

Empire Versus Democracy
The Triumph of Corporate and Military Power
Carl Boggs

Contentious Identities
Ethnic, Religious, and Nationalist Conflicts in Today's World
Daniel Chirot

The Future of Higher Education
Dan Clawson and Max Page

Waste and Consumption
Capitalism, the Environment, and the Life of Things
Simonetta Falasca-Zamponi

Rapid Climate Change
Causes, Consequences, and Solutions
Scott G. McNall

The Problem of Emotions in Societies
Jonathan H. Turner

Outsourcing the Womb
Race, Class, and Gestational Surrogacy in a Global Market
France Winddance Twine

Changing Times for Black Professionals
Adia Harvey Wingfield

How Ethical Systems Change:
Eugenics, the Final Solution, Bioethics

Sheldon Ekland-Olson
Julie Beicken
The University of Texas at Austin

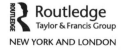
NEW YORK AND LONDON

First published 2012
by Routledge
711 Third Avenue, New York, NY 10017

Simultaneously published in the UK
by Routledge
2 Park Square, Milton Park, Abingdon, Oxon OX14 4RN

Routledge is an imprint of the Taylor & Francis Group, an informa business

Library of Congress Cataloging in Publication Date
Ekland-Olson, Sheldon, 1944–
How ethical systems change : eugenics, the final solution, bioethics / Sheldon Ekland-Olson, Julie Beicken.
p. cm. — (Framing 21st century social issues)
1. Eugenics—Moral and ethical aspects. 2. Bioethics. I. Beicken, Julie. II. Title.
HQ751.E45 2011
176—dc23
2011033062

ISBN13: 978-0-415-50162-0 (pbk)
ISBN13: 978-0-203-13156-5 (ebk)

Typeset in Garamond and Gill Sans
by EvS Communication Networx, Inc.

Printed and bound in the United States of America on acid-free paper.

University Readers (www.universityreaders.com): Since 1992, University Readers has been a leading custom publishing service, providing reasonably priced, copyright-cleared, course packs, custom textbooks, and custom publishing services in print and digital formats to thousands of professors nationwide. The Routledge Custom Gateway provides easy access to thousands of readings from hundreds of books and articles via an online library. The partnership of University Readers and Routledge brings custom publishing expertise and deep academic content together to help professors create perfect course materials that is affordable for students.

Contents

~~~~~~~~

Series Foreword

The world in the early 21st century is beset with problems—a troubled economy, global warming, oil spills, religious and national conflict, poverty, HIV, health problems associated with sedentary lifestyles. Virtually no nation is exempt, and everyone, even in affluent countries, feels the impact of these global issues.

Since its inception in the 19th century, sociology has been the academic discipline dedicated to analyzing social problems. It is still so today. Sociologists offer not only diagnoses; they glimpse solutions, which they then offer to policy makers and citizens who work for a better world. Sociology played a major role in the civil rights movement during the 1960s in helping us to understand racial inequalities and prejudice, and it can play a major role today as we grapple with old and new issues.

This series builds on the giants of sociology, such as Weber, Durkheim, Marx, Parsons, Mills. It uses their frames, and newer ones, to focus on particular issues of contemporary concern. These books are about the nuts and bolts of social problems, but they are equally about the frames through which we analyze these problems. It is clear by now that there is no single correct way to view the world, but only paradigms, models, which function as lenses through which we peer. For example, in analyzing oil spills and environmental pollution, we can use a frame that views such outcomes as unfortunate results of a reasonable effort to harvest fossil fuels. "Drill, baby, drill" sometimes involves certain costs as pipelines rupture and oil spews forth. Or we could analyze these environmental crises as inevitable outcomes of our effort to dominate nature in the interest of profit. The first frame would solve oil spills with better environmental protection measures and clean-ups, while the second frame would attempt to prevent them altogether, perhaps shifting away from the use of petroleum and natural gas and toward alternative energies that are "green."

These books introduce various frames such as these for viewing social problems. They also highlight debates between social scientists who frame problems differently. The books suggest solutions, both on the macro and micro levels. That is, they suggest what new policies might entail, and they also identify ways in which people, from the ground level, can work toward a better world, changing themselves and their lives and families and providing models of change for others.

Readers do not need an extensive background in academic sociology to benefit from these books. Each book is student-friendly in that we provide glossaries of terms for the uninitiated that are keyed to bolded terms in the text. Each chapter ends with questions for further thought and discussion. The level of each book is accessible to undergraduate students, even as these books offer sophisticated and innovative analyses.

Sheldon Ekland-Olson and his coauthors offer a fascinating four-volume analysis of the evolution of moral, ethical, and legal systems. In each volume, three themes reappear: there are important links between advances in science, technology, and evolving moral, ethical, and legal thinking; crystallizing events clarify issues and motivate reform; and boundaries of social worth are drawn when protecting and supporting life and when resolving dilemmas where the protection of life clashes with the alleviation of suffering.

In this book, Ekland-Olson and Julie Beicken trace how eugenic laws mandating that unfit individuals be prevented from having children were grounded in Darwin's theory of evolution and eventually legitimized by the U.S. Supreme Court. The U.S. eugenic legal template was used by Nazi Germany to implement their own eugenic sterilization program, and, by extension, medical experiments, practices of euthanasia, and eventually the Final Solution. Dramatic evidence of four similarly legitimized medical experiments in the United States following World War II eventually resulted in a thoroughgoing bioethics movement, grounded in principles of autonomy, beneficence, and justice.

Preface

❦

Moral systems evolve; on this there is substantial evidence. In this volume, the story begins with a broad-based social movement, led in the United States by a loosely connected network of well-educated, prosperous, elite activists. They were convinced that the ideas of Charles Darwin applied to the strength and survival of society as well as to individual species. They aimed to advance and protect society by limiting, and in the end eliminating, the feeble-minded and others judged to be unfit parasites.

Their efforts came to focus on a model mandatory sterilization law, based on what had come to be known as eugenics. As often happens, broad-based success of the eugenics movement was rooted in small, localized events. Three friends and professional colleagues in Virginia crafted a mandatory sterilization law, based on the model eugenics statute. To ensure the law's legitimacy and to protect themselves from legal repercussions, they identified a young woman they judged to be feeble-minded. They also determined that this woman's mother was feeble-minded, and that she was herself the mother of a feeble-minded daughter. In an abbreviated hearing a committee ordered that she be sterilized. In legal proceedings that followed, the colluding friends appealed their own actions to the Supreme Court, where Oliver Wendell Holmes, writing for the majority, found that three generations of imbeciles were enough. The woman was sterilized and the floodgates of mandatory sterilization across the nation for persons judged to be an unfit drain on society were opened.

Others were watching. Some six years after the Supreme Court released its decision, the newly installed government of Adolph Hitler adapted the now legitimized U.S. model statute to conditions in Germany. This German eugenics statute was the first step in what turned out to be the Final Solution. Once the soul-searing tragedies of Nazi atrocities came to light, civil and human rights movements were energized to seek a more inclusive sense of social worth. From these movements came increased protections of individual autonomy and refinements in how we thought about life and death decisions, including medical experimentation involving humans, abortion, assisted dying, and capital punishment.

1: What Lies Ahead

T he discussion in the following chapters is taken from a more detailed treatment in *Who Lives, Who Dies, Who Decides?* (Ekland-Olson 2012). The focus is upon two deeply important moral imperatives: Life is sacred and should be protected. Suffering, once detected, should be alleviated. We ask one question: How do we go about justifying the violation of these deeply important, perhaps universal, moral imperatives, while holding tightly to their importance?

The short answer is this: With empathy and logic we draw boundaries and resolve dilemmas. From time to time science, technology, and **crystallizing events** disturb, clarify, and inform existing understandings, calling for new resolutions of dilemmas and definitions of life's protective boundaries. In this manner moral systems evolve. They do so along a jagged and often contentious path.

In the next chapter, we find Charles Darwin's recently released findings and proposed explanations of evolution applied to the improvement of society. Darwin and those exploring the implications of his ideas saw some lives as more worthy of protection and support than others. They also saw social welfare programs as stalling evolution by disrupting the natural selection process. Feeble-minded and other unfit persons were likened to parasites and useless eaters. They were said to detract from and perhaps endanger the communities in which they lived. *LIFE* could and should be protected by minimizing their presence. Preventing the creation of life among these less worthy persons would not only protect *LIFE*, it would also minimize suffering.

Well-educated and influential moral entrepreneurs advanced the cause of what came to be called the eugenics movement through a loosely connected network of organizations. One was the Eugenics Record Office in Cold Spring Harbor, located some forty miles outside New York City on Long Island. One person leading the charge was a young former schoolteacher, Harry Laughlin. Laughlin spent the better part of his life carefully drafting a model statute designed to yield a uniform national policy of coercive sterilization. Using Laughlin's template, laws were crafted and a contrived trial developed which eventually wound its way to the U.S. Supreme Court. Oliver Wendell Holmes, himself a proponent of minimizing the lives of those deemed less worthy, wrote the Supreme Court opinion in *Buck v. Bell*, famously stating,

> It is better for all the world, if instead of waiting to execute **degenerate** offspring for crime, or to let them starve for their imbecility, society can prevent those who

are manifestly unfit from continuing their kind. The principle that sustains compulsory vaccination is broad enough to cover cutting the Fallopian tubes. Three generations of **imbeciles** are enough.

Much followed from this dramatic decision. In the end, the government of Adolf Hitler, borrowing heavily from Laughlin's template, legitimized by the Supreme Court, expanded Holmes' rationale to limit, manipulate, and end the lives of persons deemed less worthy. From this beginning, the Final Solution was built. When the soul-searing consequences flowing from this exclusionary framework came to light, a counter movement to secure more inclusive human and civil rights was energized.

Actions taken by the Nazis were barbarian and extreme. They had progressed step by little step. Some saw similar steps being taken in the United States. Two and a half decades after the Nuremberg Trials, four crystallizing events underscored these fears. The first was the revelation that physicians and scientists were radiating cancer patients in Ohio and other places not to cure cancer but to learn what happened to the human body in the event of an atomic bomb attack. Within months another news story chronicled how other medical researchers were feeding feces to retarded children to learn more about the causes and cures of hepatitis. Yet another group of scientists and physicians, aiming to protect the integrity of their study, were found refusing treatment, known to be effective, to men suffering from syphilis. Finally, it was revealed that physicians and scientists were experimenting with recently aborted, soon-to-die, but still living fetuses to secure additional knowledge about fetal development. In each instance lives deemed less worthy were used to benefit others considered more worthy of protection and support.

When these studies came to light, parallels to the Nuremberg trial of 23 German doctors following World War II were too clear to miss. The stage was set for federal legislation "to identify basic ethical principles." Principles were proposed and adopted. New boundaries of protected life and tolerable suffering were developed. New priorities were set for resolving dilemmas. In the process a moral system evolved.

II: An Exclusionary Movement Is Born

~~~~~~~~~~~~~~~~~~

In the aftermath of World II, the frightening consequences that an exclusionary mindset might yield became glaringly apparent. The soul-searing discovery of Nazi atrocities precipitated a broad-scale effort to clarify universal human rights and refine long-neglected civil rights. The goal was to reshape the boundaries of protected life in a more inclusive fashion. At the same time, stunning scientific discoveries produced new insights into life at the molecular level, yielding a flood of life-prolonging medical procedures and technologies. This biological revolution, with accompanying experiments, also raised questions about the protected boundaries of life, many not previously encountered.

Taken together, these dramatic cultural, scientific, and technological shifts restructured our sense of where the protective boundaries of life should be drawn. Efforts emerged to clarify the dignity and **autonomy** of the individual and to untangle the knotty problem of whether all human life, and all moments in life, are equally worthy of living, protecting, and prolonging. The consequent debates, which had been brewing for years, were accompanied by significant controversy.

Some Lives are More Worthy Than Others

The story of Nazi atrocities is often told. Only more recently has it been linked to the broadly influential framework of "applied biology" shared with colleagues in the United States as well as other European and Scandinavian countries. Important statutes and court cases in the United States predated and served as templates for the National Socialist government's exclusionary laws, defining some lives more worthy of support and protection than others. These templates were grounded in a framework that came to be known as eugenics (Barrett and Kurzman 2004; Black 2003; Kevles 1985; Kühl 1994; Stern 2005).

The eugenics movement was in many ways an embodiment of progressive thought, a purposeful attempt to improve the quality of life based on the belief that science provided an objective basis for moving toward a better future (Rogers 1982). The list of progressive movements "cross-infected" with eugenics thought included child welfare, prison reform, mental and public health, immigration rights, birth control, educational reform, and the priorities of numerous charitable foundations. Additionally, eugenics was not the intellectual property of a single political persuasion.

> Conservatives employed eugenic arguments to justify restrictions on birth control, suffrage, divorce, and women's educational and professional opportunities, while social radicals employed other eugenic arguments to assail them ... Most defended capitalism, whereas others argued that only in a classless society would it be possible to separate the genetic wheat from the chaff.
>
> (Paul 1995: 21)

Early seeds for eugenics came in the writings of an economist turned demographer, Thomas Malthus. As the 18th century drew to a close, Malthus wrote a brief but influential pamphlet: *An Essay on the Principle of Population—as it Affects the Future Improvement of Society.* His argument was simple. Humans need food, they enjoy sex, and sex produces offspring. Left unchecked, the population will grow geometrically, but the food supply will grow arithmetically. Shortages will ensue. These shortages will be differentially felt. Families should have no more children than they can support. Otherwise, they produce an unfair burden on society.

Thomas Malthus died in 1834 in Bath England. A second edition of his essay was published in 1836. Around this time, Charles Darwin, not yet thirty years old and just returned from his circumnavigation of the globe on the *Beagle*, began what he called his systematic inquiry. According to Darwin's own account, Malthus provided important theoretical grounding for his work.

> I happened to read for amusement Malthus on Population, and being well prepared to appreciate the struggle for existence which everywhere goes on from long-continued observation of the habits of animals and plants, it at once struck me that under these circumstances favourable variations would tend to be preserved, and unfavourable ones to be destroyed. The results of this would be the formation of a new species. Here, then I had at last got a theory by which to work.
>
> (1876: 47)

It would be some twenty years until *Origin of the Species* was published, but Darwin's paradigm-shifting *magnum opus* had begun. The international eugenics movement built itself on the parsimonious foundation of demography, natural selection, survival of the fittest, and policies directed at assisting Nature's selection process for the good of the whole. Governmental intrusion into the lives of individuals was justified through reference to the greater common good. Persons were categorized as productive contributors or parasitic degenerates on the basis of inherited traits. Degenerates weakened society. Their numbers should be limited.

Eugenics Becomes a Duty

In the early formative years of eugenics, no one was more important than the coiner of the term, Fancis Galton. Relying on his knowledge of animal husbandry, Galton was firm in his belief that statistical analysis of carefully gathered data yielded important insights. He was convinced that the means could be found to give "the more suitable races or strains of blood a better chance of prevailing speedily over the less suitable" (1908: 25). These means, while imperfect, were more humane than the brutal processes of natural selection. Duty and virtue thus intermixed with utilitarian calculations. In one of his frequently cited, self-reflective passages, Galton noted:

> Man is gifted with pity and other kindly feelings; he has also the power of preventing many kinds of suffering. I conceive it to fall well within his province to replace Natural Selection by other processes that are more merciful and not less effective.
>
> (1908: 323)

To alleviate or avoid suffering, life should be manipulated. Intrigued by his cousin Charles Darwin's writings, Galton began gathering data on determinants of success for persons considered luminaries of their times. He meticulously analyzed these data with statistical techniques he was then developing; techniques he refined with Karl Pearson, the British mathematician credited with establishing the field of statistics.

At the time, Galton's and Pearson's statistical techniques, still very much in use today, were revolutionary innovations aimed at discovering patterns in otherwise uncertain matters. They captured the attention of the world's best minds. Not only was the emerging field of eugenics acceptable, but thanks in large measure to the works of Darwin, Galton, and Pearson, eugenics also became compelling and respected among the intelligentsia.

Galton released an early version of his statistical study of luminaries in *Macmillan's Magazine* in 1865, and then in more detail in *Hereditary Genius* in 1869. With the appropriately cautionary notes of a conscientious scientist, he was bold in his assertions:

> I propose to show in this book that a man's natural abilities are derived by inheritance, under exactly the same limitations as are the form and physical features of the whole organic world ... I shall show that the social agencies of an ordinary character, whose influences are little suspected, are at this moment working towards the degradation of human nature, and that others are working towards its improvement. I conclude that each generation has enormous power over the natural gifts of those that follow, and maintain that it is a duty we owe to humanity to investigate the range of that power, and to exercise it in a way that, without being unwise towards ourselves, shall be most advantageous to future inhabitants of the earth.
>
> (1869: 11)

In this introductory paragraph, Galton the scientist became Galton the policy advocate.

It is one thing to assert, "man's natural abilities are derived by inheritance." It is quite another to assert that little suspected influences are working towards "the degradation of human nature, and that others are working towards its improvement," that we have "enormous power" to influence the make-up of society, and that it is a duty owed to humanity to ensure these influences "shall be most advantageous to future inhabitants of the earth."

Embedded in these latter statements is the idea that boundaries between more and less valuable life can and should be drawn. For Francis Galton and many scientists and politicians paying attention, some lives were more worthy of cultivation, protection and support than others. With this rationale, eugenics the scientific investigation became eugenics the progressive social movement.

Galton continued his work and in 1883 elaborated further on what he had in mind, coining and explaining a term for the enterprise. He wanted a word "to express the science of improving stock," a word "equally applicable to men, brutes, and plants." The term eugenics worked. It came from the Greek eugenes: "good in stock, hereditarily endowed with noble qualities." For Galton, the idea of improving the stock was not limited to judicious mating, but included "all influences that tend in however remote a degree to give to the more suitable races or strains of blood a better chance of prevailing speedily over the less suitable than they otherwise would have had" (Galton 1883: 17, fn1). The practical implications of exclusionary differential worth were beginning to grow.

While early formal membership in eugenic associations was estimated to be less than 2,000 in both Britain and the United States, there were a large number of small chapters of these associations and the message was spreading. Eventually, loosely defined networks of individuals and organizations provided a semblance of common ideological footing and coherence for the eugenics movement. Karl Pearson is said to have "exulted" to Francis Galton, in 1907, "You would be amused to hear how general is now the use of your word *Eugenics*! I hear most respectable middle-class matrons saying if children are weakly, 'Ah that was not a eugenic marriage!'" (quoted in Kevles 1985: 57). By 1910 eugenics had become one of the most frequently cited topics in the *Readers Guide to Periodical Literature* (Kevles 1985; Reilly 1991).

At the turn of the century, Galton was asked by the Anthropological Institute in London to deliver a lecture on his ideas. He titled his discussion, "The Possible Improvement of the Human Breed, Under the Existing Conditions of Law and Sentiment." Clearer understanding through data collection and analysis had taken place since his earlier works.

> The faculties of future generations will necessarily be distributed according to the laws of heredity, whose statistical effects are no longer vague, for they are measured and expressed in formulae. We cannot doubt the existence of a great power ready

to hand and capable of being directed with vast benefit as soon as we shall have learnt to understand and to apply it. To no nation is a high human breed more necessary than to our own, for we plant our stock all over the world and lay the foundation of the dispositions and capacities of future millions of the human race.

(Galton 1901)

There were boundaries to be drawn between more and less valuable forms of life, and "our" stock was better than "theirs."

In this same talk, Galton noted that the methods for "augmentation of the favored stock" might vary. Choices would have to be made. For Galton the statistician, naturalist, and policy advocate, some measures were better than others.

The possibility of improving the race of a nation depends on the power of increasing the productivity of the best stock. This is far more important than that of repressing the productivity of the worst. They both raise the average, the latter by reducing the undesirables, the former by increasing those who will become the lights of the nation. It is therefore all important to prove that favour to selected individuals might so increase their productivity as to warrant the expenditure in money and care that would be necessitated.

(Galton 1901)

These two options would find different homes. Repression of undesirables, or what came to be called **negative eugenics**, would take deepest root and become most fully developed in the United States, Canada, Scandinavia, and Germany. **Positive eugenics**, or what might be called in later parlance affirmative action for the advantaged, would become the policy of choice among eugenic advocates in Great Britain.

Throughout the closing decades of the 19th century, a Malthusian future was looming. Resources were strained by a severe depression. Prosperous citizens were having children at or just below replacement levels. Among the less prosperous and newly arrived immigrants, those least able to support their children, offspring were arriving at much higher rates. To make matters worse, society was providing a safety net for these less advantaged persons. This weakened the natural winnowing that would otherwise occur. Eugenicists criticized "indiscriminate benevolence" for the poor as it produced artificially long life spans for the unfit. If left unchecked, these higher birth rates and artificially reduced death rates among society's least capable could mean only one thing—the slow but sure degrading of the population. Survival of a thriving prosperous society was at stake (Popenoe and Johnson 1918).

The negative eugenic argument was attractively simple. Wouldn't it be better to have a society enriched by those who are productive, healthy, emotionally stable, and smart than one stifled by degenerate, feeble-minded, disabled and criminal citizens? To protect *LIFE* writ large, the lives of those less worthy should be reduced in number.

Knowing now that this argument led to the Final Solution, it is almost automatic to be repulsed by the proposed journey.

How did well-educated individuals, schooled in the healing arts and the rigors and self-correcting mechanisms of science, supported by prominent, well endowed philanthropic foundations whose mission it was to make society better, go so badly wrong? Step by little step in a climate of fear that *LIFE* needed protection seems to be the answer. A loosely connected network of individuals and organizations, dedicated to the eugenics cause, began to chart the course toward what they saw as a more secure future (Beicken 2009).

A Base of Operation

The framing message and assumption of eugenics was differential worth. Some lives were more worthy of support and protection than others. There was research to be done, the fruits of which could be used for the betterment of all. Pioneering efforts took root in the American Breeders' Association, The American Eugenics Society, The Galton Society, the Race Betterment Foundation, and the Human Betterment Foundation (Allen 1986; Kevles 1985). No organization, however, was more important as an early base of operation than the Station for the Experimental Study of Evolution (SESE) and the Eugenics Record Office (ERO) at Cold Spring Harbor, Long Island, New York.

The SESE and ERO were launched through the efforts of a young entrepreneurial professor, Charles Benedict Davenport. Davenport, a biologist with mathematical training, received his PhD in 1892 from Harvard. His interests led him to the works of Galton, Pearson, and Mendel. He was eventually appointed to the editorial board of Pearson's journal, *Biometrika*. Reviewing articles for this newly founded journal put him in touch with other like-minded scholars reporting their research on a wide range of related topics.

The empirical methods taking hold in biology at the time, especially those exploring the links between the ideas of Mendel and Darwin's evolutionary theories, needed a home. Davenport was convinced of the importance of this enterprise, noting the parallels between improving the quality of thoroughbred horses, hogs, cattle and sheep and the vitality and strength of the human population. It was a promising, exciting enterprise, well worth pursuing.

While teaching at Harvard and then at the University of Chicago, Davenport began seeking funds to establish an independent laboratory. He had taught at a small summer institute on the northwestern shore of Long Island and thought it would be an ideal location for the operation he had in mind. He knew also that the philanthropic Carnegie Institution of Washington (CIW) had just been founded and that their funding priorities coincided with his interests.

Through an influential banker friend in Chicago, Davenport submitted a funding proposal aimed at exploring "the analytic and experimental study of the cause of specific differentiation—of race change" (Allen 1986: 229). The proposal was turned down. Davenport had failed to spell out and the CIW had failed to recognize the broader implications of what he had in mind. The CIW was most interested in proposals that would have broad-based practical impact as well as in funding researchers and organizations that would coordinate efforts toward a common goal.

As young researchers often do, Davenport learned of this assessment and CIW's predisposition to broad-based practical projects that worked across disciplines. He rewrote his proposal and resubmitted. In December of 1903 he was awarded a grant with commitments "to continue indefinitely, or for a long time." The Station for the Experimental Study of Evolution was born.

As work moved forward, Davenport formed an alliance with the American Breeders Association (ABA) created in St. Louis, Missouri, the same year funding for the Station for the Experimental Study of Evolution was secured. At their first meeting, Davenport was elected to the ABA oversight committee and was instrumental in establishing the Eugenics Committee. This committee was charged, in the hereditary parlance of the day, to "devise methods of recording the values of the blood of individuals, families, people and races" with the overarching purpose of emphasizing "the value of superior blood and the menace to society of inferior blood" (Black 2003: 39).

It became increasingly clear that carefully kept records and a repository for data were essential to the research being pursued. Plans began almost immediately to add such capacity, but again funding was needed. In testament to the strength of weak ties (Granovetter 1983; Snow, Zurcher, and Ekland-Olson 1980) and the importance of a tenacious entrepreneurial spirit for the success of any social movement, Davenport knew that railroad magnate, Edward Henry Harriman, had recently died and had left control of his fortune to his wife, Mary Harriman. He knew also that the widow's daughter had been a student of his some three years earlier in the summer program at Cold Spring Harbor.

He wrote Mrs. Harriman, who was distributing a portion of her fortune through a philanthropic foundation devoted to providing individuals an opportunity to become "more efficient members of society." Harriman placed special emphasis on the use of scientific principles to secure a rational, orderly society (Allen 1986: 234). What better match could there be than with the Station for the Experimental Study of Evolution? Renewing their acquaintance and noting his admiration for her philanthropic endeavors, Davenport suggested that the newly launched endeavor at Cold Spring Harbor would be a good fit for the priorities of the Harriman Foundation.

Of all the letters Mary Harriman received, reportedly some six thousand, Davenport's was one that stood out. Davenport and Harriman gathered for subsequent conversations to discuss what he had in mind and how it matched the goals of the Foundation. Convinced this was the case, Harriman made a financial commitment to Davenport that resulted in the creation of the Eugenics Record Office. Harry Laughlin, a former teacher and school superintendent from Missouri who had become acquainted with Davenport through the American Breeders Association (ABA) was appointed to head up the ERO.

Funding from the Carnegie Institute of Washington and the Harriman Foundation provided much needed resources as well as added credibility and a place at the table with society's elite for the fledging enterprise. The operation at Cold Spring Harbor was an operation to be taken seriously. It soon became "a meeting place for eugenicists, a repository for eugenics records, a clearinghouse for eugenics information and propaganda, a platform from which popular eugenic campaigns could be launched, and a home for several eugenical publications." The ERO, in short, "became a nerve center for the eugenics movement as a whole" (Allen 1986: 226).

From Cold Spring Harbor and the eventual expansion of related operations across the country, the eugenics movement evolved. Conferences were held, studies conducted, papers and books written, speeches given, sermons delivered, laws crafted and passed. Contrived lawsuits were filed, expert testimony was provided, and Supreme Court decisions were produced. It would be a long-lasting, far-reaching, and, in the end, quite troubling legacy.

Framing the Agenda

The Cold Spring Harbor operation worked hand-in-hand with the American Breeders Association (Kimmelman 1983). Davenport had been elected to the ABA oversight committee, and in 1906 he helped establish a Eugenics Committee. The committee's charge was to develop methods for mapping traits of families, individuals and races, with the underlying assumption that some "blood lines" were beneficial and some detrimental to the health of society. Early human eugenics in the United States grew largely from the efforts of this ABA committee. Its membership was luminary.

David Starr Jordan, the first president of Stanford University, agreed to serve as the committee's chair. His colleagues on the committee included Alexander Graham Bell and Luther Burbank. As indicated in a membership pamphlet put out by the ABA, their purpose was to advance the "interests of the Association that relate to human improvement by a better selection of marriage mates and the control of the reproduction of defective classes" (Beicken 2009: 512–15). Much of the ABA's human eugenics initiative transferred to Cold Spring Harbor. Shortly after Harry Laughlin took the superintendent's job at the ERO, the task of producing an early report for Jordan's committee became his responsibility.

Jordan had long-standing interests in these matters. As a young professor in Indiana, he had become acquainted with Oscar McCulloch, the minister of the Indianapolis Congregational Church. A captivating orator and central figure in the social gospel and charity reform movements of the time, Reverend McCulloch was dedicated to improving the condition of man. He had been responsible for establishing numerous charitable organizations in the Indianapolis area. He sensed a degradation of society, spoke frequently of this in his sermons, and was a vocal advocate for change (Weeks 1976).

Among his many causes, McCulloch was a frequent and outspoken critic of the injustices of capital punishment, advocating as well for a more humane prison system modeled after a recently constructed reformatory in Elmira, New York. Thanks to his efforts and influence, Indiana was the first state to establish a reformatory for women and girls. A parallel institution for men would soon follow. These reformatories would become the site of pioneering mandatory sterilization efforts.

Reverend McCulloch was impressed by Galton's research. He was drawn also to Richard Dugdale's study of an extended family in New York, first published in 1877, *"The Jukes" A Study in Crime, Pauperism, Disease and Heredity.* It provided, McCulloch believed, important insights into both cause and remedy of degenerate persons who so troubled and damaged the society he aimed to improve. There were stories of a similarly situated family involved in crime and socially degrading behavior throughout Indiana. McCulloch decided to investigate.

He would later recall his first contact with the Ishmaels in the fall of 1877:

> There were gathered in one room, without fire, an old blind woman, a man, his wife and one child, his sister and two children. A half-bed was all the furnishing. No chair, table, or cooking utensils. I provided for their immediate wants, and then looked into the records of the township trustee.
>
> (McCulloch 1891: 2)

From this initial meeting, McCulloch expanded his investigation over the next decade, eventually including over two hundred and fifty families connected through an extended familial network, thirty of which were investigated in greater depth. Eleven years after his initial contact, in 1888, McCulloch presented his findings, at a National Conference of Charities and Corrections, held in Buffalo, New York, introducing the world to *The Tribe of Ishmael: A Study of Social Degradation.*

He began with an analogy. There were parallels, McCulloch noted, between this tribe and a small, free-swimming, parasitic crustacean, then being studied by a University of Chicago professor, Ray Lankaster (1880). Soon after birth, "an irresistible hereditary tendency seizes upon it." It attaches to a crab, losing in the process "the characteristics of the higher class, and becomes degraded in form and function." This parasitic behavior is transmitted to its offspring and it stands "in nature as a type of degradation through parasitism, or pauperism."

With the parasitic crustacean imagery in place, McCulloch continued. "I propose to trace the history of similar degradation in man. It is no pleasant study, but it may be relied upon as fact. It is no isolated case. It is not peculiar to Indiana." Nearing the end of his presentation, Reverend McCulloch underscored his analogy between those he had studied and the parasitic crustacean.

> They are a decaying stock; they can no longer live self-dependent. The children reappear with the old basket. The girl begins the life of prostitution, and is soon seen with her own illegitimate child. The young of the Sacculina at first have the Nauplius form common to their order. Then the force of inherited parasitism compels them to fasten themselves to the hermit crab. The free-swimming legs and the disused organs disappear. So we have the same in the pauper. Self–help disappears. All the organs and powers that belong to the free life disappear, and there are left only the tendency to parasitism and the debasement of the reproductive tendency.
>
> (1891: 8)

Like parasites, the Tribe of Ishmael, from one generation to the next, sucked nutrients from society and in the process became useless dependents.

This energy sapping degradation, McCulloch concluded, was hereditary. It was also pushed along by misplaced charity. "The so-called charitable people who give to begging children and women with baskets have a vast sin to answer for ... So-called charity joins public relief in producing still-born children, raising prostitutes, and educating criminals" (McCulloch 1891: 8). For the moment, this preacher of the social gospel, this organizer of charitable organizations and innovative reformatories had apparently become disenchanted with a New Testament account of the final judgment involving those who were charitable and those who were not (Book of Matthew 25: 34–45).

He closed his presentation with a final admonition. "What can we do? First, we must close up official out-door relief. Second we must check private and indiscriminate benevolence, or charity, falsely so-called. Third, we must get hold of the children." Three years after presenting his findings, Oscar McCulloch, the minister, researcher, and social reformer had become president of the National Conference of Charities and Corrections. Shortly thereafter, at the age of forty-eight, he died an untimely death from his inherited Hodgkin's Disease (Weeks 1976).

McCulloch's dehumanizing parasitic characterization of the Tribe of Ishmael, and those of the same ilk was longer lasting and widely shared. In 1902, a decade after McCulloch's death, the president of what is today known as the American Association on Intellectual and Developmental Disabilities, M. W. Barr, made another presentation to the National Conference of Charities and Corrections. His topic: "The Imbecile and Epileptic Versus the Tax-Payer and the Community." His conclusion: "[O]f all dependent classes there are none that drain so entirely the social and financial life of the body politic as the imbecile, unless it be its close associate, the epileptic" (Barr quoted in Wolfensberger 1975: 34).

Branching Out

By the time Reverend McCulloch's parishioner, David Starr Jordan, accepted his appointment as chair of the American Breeders Association's committee, charged with mapping traits beneficial or detrimental to the health of society, he had become a well-known academic. He resigned as president of Indiana University to become Leland Stanford Junior University's (now, Stanford University) first president the same year Oscar McCulloch died. Armed with McCulloch's, sermons, research and policy conclusions, as well as his own work and the writings of other prominent academicians, Jordan became a linchpin for the eugenic movement on the west coast.

His position and academic standing made him attractive on the lecture circuit, both nationally and internationally. In 1898, ten years after Oscar McCulloch had introduced the world to the Tribe of Ishmael, he collected many of his writings in *Foot-Notes to Evolution: A Series of Popular Addresses on the Evolution of Life,* and published them along with supplemental essays by three of his colleagues at Stanford and the University of Pennsylvania. The next year, he gave a widely debated speech at Stanford, *The Blood of a Nation: A Study of the Decay of Races Through the Survival of the Unfit,* which was eventually published in 1902 and then reprinted by the American Unitarian Association in 1907 along with a related speech he delivered in Philadelphia at ceremonies celebrating the two-hundredth anniversary of the birth of Benjamin Franklin (Jordan 1907).

By this time Jordan's eugenics position had solidified. In *Blood of a Nation* he wrote,

> For a race of men or a herd of cattle are governed by the same laws of selection ... In selective breeding ... it is possible, with a little attention to produce wonderful changes for the better.... To select for posterity those individuals which best meet our needs or please our fancy, and to destroy those with unfavorable qualities, is the function of artificial selection.
>
> (Jordan 1902: 12)

President Jordan's perspective had been further shaped by several visits he made to the Village of Aosta, located in a sparsely populated, scenic, alpine valley not far from majestic Mont Blanc, where Italy, France, and Switzerland converge. There he had observed a community of "cretins." Later, in his autobiography, he would recall this community as "feeble little people with uncanny voices, silly faces, and sickening smiles, incapable of taking care of themselves" (Jordan 1922: 314). By 1910 this community had all but died out as a result of segregation in an asylum where the Church would neither condone marriage, nor permit child bearing. Jordan drew upon this lesson of selective breeding through enforced segregation in the years just ahead.

With this background, prominence, and perspective, Stanford's president accepted the request from the American Breeders Association and the Eugenics Record Office to develop policy recommendations for human eugenics. In 1911 Jordan began work with Harry Laughlin on a study, funded in part by the Carnegie Institution, to explore the "best practical means for cutting off the defective germ-plasm in the human population." The eugenics movement was gaining momentum in a now nationwide network of connections.

It was also redefining itself and broadening its mission. The American Breeders Association changed its name to the American Genetics Association. Its official publication, *American Breeders Magazine*, became the *Journal of Heredity*. A former Stanford student of Jordan's, Paul Popenoe, was appointed as its editor.

The Criteria for Exclusion

At this time, understandings of heredity were primitive at best. The structure of DNA and genetic markers was nowhere on the horizon. Instead, researchers continued to rely on the distribution of traits as revealed in pedigree studies of familial networks such as studies of the Jukes and the Ishmaels produced by Dugdale and McCulloch.

A common thread in these family studies was how to separate those unfit, from those worthy and contributing. To better define these boundaries, Davenport published *The Trait Book* (1912), a detailed listing of individual characteristics, predispositions and behavioral tendencies. In it, he devised guidelines for field observations, pedigree charts, and surveys. These were widely distributed to physicians, teachers, social workers, and parents. Classification schemes to organize the data were devised. The feeble-minded, degenerate, perverts, **morons**, imbeciles, epileptics, and paupers were defined as lives less worthy. They were to be identified, isolated, minimized and, if possible, eliminated.

While definitions of exclusionary boundaries remained loose and subject to wide interpretation among field workers, continuing attempts were made to refine definitions and data gathering techniques. Training was provided before sending persons, mainly women, into the field to observe and identify manifestations of the defined traits. Quantitative intelligence testing, being developed in France at the time, was adapted to further assist these efforts.

As the Cold Spring Harbor operation was getting off the ground, French psychologists Alfred Binet and Theodore Simon designed the **Simon-Binet Scale** between 1905 and 1908. A few years later Lewis Terman, a Stanford professor and colleague of David Starr Jordan, offered a modified version of the test, known as the Stanford-Binet test. A close associate of Charles Davenport and the ERO, Henry Goddard, translated the work of Binet and Simon into English in 1908 and introduced benchmarks to identify "morons," persons with marginal intelligence, from "imbeciles" (one category lower), and "**idiots**" (two categories lower).

Goddard was the director of the research laboratory at the Vineland Training School for Feebleminded Girls and Boys in New Jersey. He believed at the time that such children would grow up to have higher fertility rates than others and thus advocated tight controls on their abilities to have children. As part of the growing network of eugenic cooperation, Goddard routinely made his patients available for family pedigree tracing and assessment and was intimately involved in writing reports for the ERO.

In one of these reports Goddard reviewed his impressions of the quality of the data being collected:

> The field worker goes out as the superintendent's personal representative with a letter recommending her [females were seen as most effective interviewers] and urging the parents, for the sake of the child, to tell all they possibly can, and to send her to other relatives or to any one who may be able to give information, which may be used to help their child, or some one's child. The response has been full, free, and hearty. Parents do all in their power to help us get the facts. There is very rarely anything like an attempt to conceal facts that they know. Of course, many of these parents are ignorant, often feeble-minded, and cannot tell all that we should like to know. Nevertheless, by adroit questioning and cross–reference, we have been able to get what we believe to be very accurate data in a very large percentage of our cases.
>
> (Eugenics Record Office 1911: 1)

One can only speculate how these families might have responded had they known more fully that an underlying purpose of Goddard's studies was to limit the existence of persons such as themselves and families such as their own.

Whatever the response, later assessments of family pedigree studies were not kind. One particularly critical reviewer would note,

> The movement continued to amass volumes of data on families and individuals by combining equal portions of gossip, race prejudice, sloppy methods, and leaps of logic, all caulked together by elements of actual genetic knowledge to create the glitter of a genuine science.
>
> (Black 2003: 105)

Goddard himself would eventually question the validity of his conclusions along with their eugenic implications.

The early family pedigree studies of the Jukes and the Ishmaels, along with less well-publicized related research, however, were soon joined by other works, including Goddard's widely disseminated and highly influential investigation of the Kallikaks (Goddard 1912) and Aurthur Estabrook's (1916) re-examination of data on the Jukes. Armed with the experience of his work, Estabrook became an expert witness in a contrived trial involving forced sterilization of a young woman in Virginia, Carrie Buck.

The Passing of the Great Race, authored by Madison Grant in 1916, a friend and professional associate of Davenport and the ERO, also joined this growing body of academic literature. These individuals and their works played major roles as the eugenic movement continued its journey. Grant's work, widely translated, was greeted with mixed reviews. Columbia University professor and well-known anthropologist Franz Boas and his soon to become equally famous student Margaret Mead were among its most severe critics. In contrast, the work was favorably reviewed in *Science*, the journal of the American Association for the Advancement of Science (Woods 1918). Most infamously, it would be praised and used as a template by a young Adolf Hitler when he wrote *Mein Kampf* from his jail cell.

The negative eugenics movement clearly had broad reach and influence. A relatively small, loose-knit circle of colleagues, centered at the Eugenics Record Office in Cold Spring Harbor, shaped the agenda. Their aim was to establish a nationwide program of mandatory sterilization grounded in statutory law. It began with David Starr Jordan's committee and a 200-page report largely written by Harry Laughlin.

DISCUSSION QUESTIONS

1. What are the connections between the eugenic program advanced in the United States and the Nazi Holocaust? What are some of the common ideological points that bring the two together?

2. Do you think that the eugenicists' methods of gathering data were scientific? Why or why not?

3. What are the connections between scientific understanding of how the world works and policy decisions about how the world should work?

4. How does the understanding of heredity at the turn of the 20th century compare to our understanding at the turn of the 21st?

5. What are some of the policy issues that have arisen from our more recent understanding of heredity?

III: Legal Reform to Eliminate Defectives

~~~

The legal effort to justify mandatory sterilization was carefully orchestrated. It began when Harry Laughlin released a 200-page report on the "best practical means of cutting off the defective germ plasm in the American population," in February of 1914 (Eugenics Record Office, *Bulletin No. 10A* 1914; Eugenics Record Office, *Bulletin No. 10B,* 1914). Laughlin later drafted and released a model law in 1922 that grew directly from this earlier report. Many of the ideas in Laughlin's report had been presented and discussed at the First National Conference on Race Betterment, held the month prior to the release of the 1914 report in Battle Creek Michigan. Laughlin's 1922 proposal served as a template for laws enacted in the United States and was eventually upheld as Constitutional by the Supreme Court in *Buck v. Bell* in 1927. It also provided the foundation for Germany's first sterilization law enacted in 1933, shortly after Adolf Hitler came to power. In gratitude for his pioneering work, so helpful in guiding Germany's early efforts, Heidelberg University awarded Laughlin an honorary degree in 1936 for his work on "racial cleansing."

A Moral Entrepreneur Reviews the Landscape

The journey from Laughlin's 1914 report to the horrors of Nazi Germany was taken step by step over three decades. A model statute was a starting point as activists aimed to isolate degenerates and take advantage of a new surgical technique, developed for sterilizing men. Laughlin knew that a minor surgical technique, eventually known as a vasectomy, had been developed in the late 1890s by Dr. Albert Ochsner, reported in 1899 in the *Journal of the American Medical Association.* Vasectomies were seen as far more acceptable in both law and public opinion than castration. Early efforts, however, to apply this relatively simple procedure met with mixed success. For women and young girls, similarly minor sterilization procedures were yet to be developed.

A champion for the cause was needed. Harry Laughlin Stood ready and perhaps more than any other single individual became the moral and policy entrepreneur for mandatory eugenic sterilization. He began looking for lessons from others.

One lesson came from Pennsylvania, where on March 21, 1905, both houses of the legislature in Pennsylvania passed an Act for the Prevention of Idiocy. While the bill had solid support in the Pennsylvania Legislature, it had none from the state's governor, Samuel Pennypacker. Governor Pennypacker found the bill wanting on several fronts. In prescient anticipation of what many years later would be called the Georgetown Principles of **Bioethics** (Beauchamp and Childress 2001), Governor Pennypacker noted that in the bill's provisions doctor-patient trust was breached, patient autonomy was violated, **beneficence** neglected, malevolence imposed, and **justice** ignored. "To permit such an operation," the governor commented, "would be to inflict cruelty upon a helpless class of the community which the state has undertaken to protect." "A great objection is that the bill," the governor continued, "would be the beginning of experimentation upon living human beings, leading logically to results which can readily be forecasted." He disagreed with the wisdom, justice, practicality and legality of such a law. He was governor. He had veto power. A little over a week after the bill was passed, he exercised this power. History and the Nuremberg Doctors' Trials would prove Governor Pennypacker right.

The experience in Indiana two years later was different. Here the lessons learned about the dangers of degenerates from Oscar McCulloch and David Starr Jordan were first put into practice and then into law. Working with inmates in Indiana's reformatory, Dr. Harry Sharp had begun imposing vasectomies shortly after the procedure was proposed in 1899 (Ochsner 1899). Within less than a decade he had vasectomized over 200 patients. Based on his experience as Indiana Reformatory's chief surgeon, Sharp began to lobby for legal change. He had been able to perform his sterilizations without a legal statute in part because reformatories and their outcast inmates were far from the public eye. Having enabling legislation, however, would provide legal cover if needed.

In 1907 Indiana became the first state to have an involuntary sterilization law. The Indiana law was very close in word, procedure, and purpose to the law Governor Pennypacker had vetoed. This time, however, three days after passage, Governor J. Frank Hanley signed the bill into law. The law was not designed to impose punishment for any crime. Instead, its design was eugenic and its purpose public health. Discretion was granted to a committee of experts: "If, in the judgment of this committee of experts and the board of managers, procreation is inadvisable, and there is no probability of improvement of the mental and physical condition of the inmate, it shall be lawful for the surgeons to perform such operation for the prevention of procreation as shall be decided safest and most effective." Dr. Harry Sharp had argued that surgical and administrative procedures were safe, painless, fair, and positive in impact.

Predictably, persons sterilized did not always agree. Several inmates among the reported 119 men sterilized in Indiana Reformatory during the first year of the law's existence took exception and wrote letters (Stern 2007: 103) to Hanley's successor, Governor Thomas Marshall, who would soon become Woodrow Wilson's Vice President. These letters noted the perfunctory nature of the conversations leading to sterilization decisions, and asserted that whatever the law's stated eugenic purpose, its consequences were punitive and lacking in procedural safeguards. These letters found a sympathetic ear in recently elected Governor Marshall, who was not in the same political camp as Sharp, Hurty, and Hanley. The governor had previously expressed his concern that procedural safeguards for reaching eugenic decisions were almost totally lacking. He was not convinced that the law was strictly eugenic rather than punitive. It was most certainly punitive in individual consequences where persons did not desire to be sterilized.

Between March 1907, when Indiana's legislation was signed into law, and the February 1914 release of the Laughlin committee's recommendations, eleven additional states passed statutes similar to Indiana's. Nowhere did the eugenic sterilization movement take deeper root than in California, the adopted home of David Starr Jordan. The legislature enacted the state's first nonconsensual sterilization law in 1909. There was only 1 dissenting vote out of 63, and the governor signed the legislation into law. Legislation repealing the law was precipitated by a class action suit, *Madrigal v. Quilligan,* involving coerced postpartum tubal ligations of predominantly working class women of Mexican origin (see Stern 2005). Modified several times over the years, and falling into some disuse after the revealed Nazi horrors of World War II, it was not until 1979 that California's sterilization statute was finally repealed in a social climate of heightened concern over governmental intrusion into individual lives.

Framing a Legitimized Logic of Exclusion

As the eugenic movement gained momentum, current beliefs and the best available evidence suggested that the place to start was with persons housed in reformatory and penal institutions, as well as state institutions "for the insane, the feeble-minded, the epileptic, the inebriate, and the pauper classes" (the following quotes are from Eugenics Record Office Report to the Committee 1914). Laughlin and his committee recognized that not all inmates in these institutions would qualify for mandatory sterilization. The aim of mandatory sterilization was not punishment. It was a public health measure. In both "intent and phrasing the proposed sterilization law should follow the strictest eugenical motives, and should be based upon the theory that sterilization is of such consequences that it should be ordered only by due process of law and only after expert investigation."

Family pedigree studies were increasingly used to determine the potential inmates had for producing defective offspring. Laughlin's law proposed that the responsibility for determining such potential was to be given to a Eugenics Commission, composed of persons possessing expert knowledge of biology, pathology, and psychology. The head of each institution would have the responsibility of providing the Eugenics Commission with the inmate's mental and physical conditions, innate traits, personal record, family traits and history.

The eugenics examination was to be carried out on all inmates prior to their release. For those found likely to be parents of "defectives," the Eugenics Commission would report its findings to a state court, including a recommendation for the appropriate sterilizing operation. The court would then examine the evidence "allowing ample opportunity for the individual in question, or his relatives, guardian or friends to be heard." If the court concluded the individual had the potential for producing children who would "probably, because of inherited defective or anti-social traits, become a social menace or a ward of the state," the court would order the head of the institution "to cause to be performed ... in a safe and humane manner, a surgical operation of effective sterilization before his or her release or discharge."

Laughlin's committee specified these principles in what they saw as a Model Sterilization Law. Their aim was in two generations to "practically cut off the inheritance lines and consequently the further supply of that portion of the human stock now measured by the lowest and most degenerate one-tenth of the total population." A very precise schedule, complete with "Rate of Efficiency" graphs, was provided to achieve total elimination of defectives in seven decades. In rough approximation, the total number of yearly sterilizations nationwide would rise from 92,000 in 1920; to 121,000 by 1930; 158,000 by 1940; 203,000 by 1950; 260,000 by 1960; 330,000 by 1970; and 415,000 by 1980. The stakes were high. The degenerate one-tenth constituted a "growing menace" to the nation's social welfare. Legal reforms should start immediately.

Thus, the issues were framed. The Laughlin report was released in February of 1914. Six months later, Germany declared war on France and invaded Belgium. The bloody war years (1914–1918) consumed the nation's attention. The eugenics movement would have to wait. It lost steam, but did not come to a halt. It was supported by a receptive exclusionary climate.

A Receptive Exclusionary Climate

The eugenics cause was embedded in a broader cultural climate infused with an us-and-them mindset. Some lives were more worthy of protection, support and encouragement than others. As Laughlin's committee sought legitimate ways to minimize the procreation of less worthy lives, the country was working its way through a rabidly racist and xenophobic period.

Jim Crow Laws had been passed in the closing years of the 19th century. These same years saw a sharp increase in lynchings. By 1914 lynchings were tapering off but continued at historically high levels through the 1920s (see, for example, Tolnay and Beck 1995). The Ku Klux Klan, disbanded after the Civil Rights Act of 1871, was being reinvented (Chalmers 1987). In 1916 Madison Grant published his widely read and instantly reprinted book, *The Passing of the Great Race*. As noted in Chapter 2,

Grant was closely associated with colleagues at Cold Spring Harbor and the eugenics movement on both the east and west coasts. A graduate of Yale University and Columbia Law School, Grant couched his review of how demographic and migration patterns had shaped history in rhetoric that drew at once on the self-correcting methods of science and the unbending and sometimes bombastic convictions of an activist.

Instead of welcoming the homeless and tempest-tossed, the huddled masses yearning to breathe free, Grant's belief, echoing Oscar McCulloch before him, was that "altruistic ideals" and "maudlin sentimentalism" had made America an "asylum for the oppressed" who were in fact leading the country toward a "racial abyss." His book's closing lines reflected his major worry: "If the Melting Pot is allowed to boil without control and we continue to follow our national motto and deliberately blind ourselves to all 'distinctions of race, creed, or color' ..." those of Colonial descent would go the way of the "Athenian of the age of Pericles, and the Viking of the days of Rollo" (Grant 1916: 263).

The year just prior to the publication of Grant's book, *The Birth of a Nation*, a widely viewed and heroic cinematic depiction of the Ku Klux Klan, based on Thomas Dixon's book, *The Clansman*, was released. President Woodrow Wilson, Dixon's classmate at Johns Hopkins, reportedly gave it a positive review, although some suspected Dixon might have been the source of positive comments attributed to the Wilson. The recently reborn KKK made use of the film as a recruitment tool. Due to its controversial nature, showings were sometimes greeted by counterbalancing protests, movie cancellations and riots in several large cities.

In the more strictly eugenic arena, *The Black Stork* was released the same year as *The Passing of the Great Race*. Shown over the next decade, this film made a strong connection between eugenics and doing God's will. It was a dramatization of the widely publicized experiences and practices of a Chicago surgeon, Dr. Harry Haiseldon, who had allowed defective infants to die. His actions drew substantial public attention and generated both support and opposition. Reflecting the wide dissemination of family pedigree studies at the time, when asked about his practices, Haiseldon told a reporter, "What do you prefer—six days of Baby Bollinger or seventy years of the Jukes?" (Pernick 1996: 42; see also Chapter 8). Helen Keller, well known for her strong advocacy for persons with disabilities, herself a person Dr. Haiseldon might have let die as an infant, joined in support of the doctor's action. In a letter to *The New Republic*, written shortly after the publicity surrounding Haiseldon broke, Keller likened his actions to "weeding of the human garden that shows a sincere love of true life" (Keller 1915: 173–74).[1]

---

1 For a discussion of apparent contradictions in Hellen Keller's public pronouncements, see Gerdtz 2006.

Importantly, the film introduced a eugenic theme rejected by Laughlin's committee—the termination of defective lives. Mandatory sterilization to avoid the birth of "defectives" was one thing. Killing or allowing to die was quite another, even if, as the images of the film implied, the baby ascended into the waiting arms of Jesus. The underlying themes of terminating life or knowingly letting an infant die under various circumstances later became a major item of bioethical debate in the latter half of the 20th century. Regardless of the debates to come, those intimately involved in the early eugenics movement clearly thought some lives more worthy of support, protection than others. Just as clearly, they thought governmental intrusion was called for. The strength of communal life was at stake. They would, on occasion, even consider the merits of **euthanasia** for "nature's mistakes" (Kennedy 1942: 13–16).

Whatever the underlying rationale, momentum for eugenic legal reform and governmental action to protect public health was regenerated in the years following the "war to end all wars." In particular, two new and eventually highly influential organizations were launched, each rooted in an existing national network of personal relations.

Mobilizing Resources and Networks of Support

The American Eugenics Society was conceived and developed in the early 1920s. Its chief architect, Henry Fairfield Osborne, was the President of the American Museum of Natural History and a collaborator with Madison Grant on *The Passing of the Great Race*. Harry Laughlin, Madison Grant, and Harry Crampton, a well-respected evolutionary biologist, joined Osborne in his AES initiatives. AES's major focus was public education. The aim was to move beyond the dry analysis of academic publications and conferences, beyond the elite circles of the Ivy League, the University of Chicago, and Stanford, to the heartland. If the eugenics movement was to succeed, networks of support needed to expand.

County fair exhibits became a staple of this public education campaign. They came complete with flashing lights demonstrating how high birth rates among the unfit, those "born to be a burden on the rest," were degrading the nation. "Fitter family" and "better baby" contests were organized. Much like prize cows, chickens, and hogs, families and babies were judged by physical appearance, health, behavior, and intelligence. The winners were awarded medals and ribbons for demonstrating high quality breeding.

As the American Eugenics Society was getting off the ground, the Human Betterment Foundation was launched in California. Its core members included David Starr Jordan and Paul Popenoe. Connections with the ERO in New York, programs in Indiana, and the Race Betterment Foundation in Michigan were evident. In California, the wealthy citrus grower and philanthropist, Ezra Gosney provided resources making the Human Betterment Foundation perhaps the most well-funded eugenic organization in the country (Reilly 1987). In this California-based operation, resources were primarily aimed at data gathering and analysis with particular emphasis on the impact and success of compulsory sterilization. Reports from the HBF, illustrated by Gosney and Popenoe's *Sterilization for Human Betterment* (1929), were widely disseminated and discussed.

The Legal Framework Clarifies

Laughlin's initial report to the ERO was released in 1914. By 1921 eight state laws had been challenged in state and federal appellate courts. They did not fare well. All but one was overturned, either in whole or in part. This had a dampening effect on the eugenics movement, but working with a colleague in Chicago, Judge Harry Olson, Laughlin took lessons from these appellate decisions as he refined his model sterilization law.

Many of the legal issues had come up just prior to the 1914 report. One was in New Jersey, home of Goddard's Vineland Training School for Feebleminded Girls and Boys. Then governor and future president, Woodrow Wilson, had signed the new law in 1911. It authorized the sterilization of the "feeble-minded (including Morons, Imbeciles, and Idiots), epileptic, rapists, and certain criminals and other defectives" who were confined in the state's reformatories, charitable and penal institutions. An appeal was made on behalf of a young epileptic woman, Alice Smith (*Smith v. Board of Examiners of Feeble-Minded* 1913).[2] Alice had been confined in New Jersey's State Village for Epileptics since 1902. While her epilepsy was not contested, at the time of her hearing she had not had a seizure for five years. In May of 1912, armed with the recently passed law, a committee was convened to determine whether it was advisable that she be sterilized by salpingectomy. It determined that it was and so ordered. The committee's action was appealed to New Jersey's Supreme Court. Justice Garrison, on behalf of two other colleagues, rendered the court's opinion. Neither he nor his colleagues were at all convinced that the mandated sterilization of Alice Smith was either wise or legal.

They noted in specific detail the seriousness of a salpingectomy. It involved "… the incision or excision of the Fallopian tube, i.e., either cutting it off or cutting it out." Unlike a vasectomy, this procedure was "deep-seated surgery under profound and prolonged anaesthesia, and hence (involved) all of the dangers of life incident thereto,

---

2 Among other reasons, this case is interesting since later in his life, Harry Laughlin would find that he, too, was epileptic. Many critical commentators would note the irony of Laughlin's diagnosis in later years.

whether arising from the anaesthetic, from surgical shock or from the inflammation or infection incident to surgical interference." The statute's vague wording also bothered the judges, as its sterilization authority was broad enough to authorize an operation to remove any of a woman's organs essential for procreation—ovaries, fallopian tubes, and uterus.

Given this assessment, the reasons for state intervention for coercive sterilization had to be compelling. The stated motivating reason: public health. For these three New Jersey judges, this was a "novel" rationale, one that asserted the "theoretical improvement of society by destroying the function of procreation in certain of its members who are not malefactors against its laws." Similar to concerns Governor Pennypacker had articulated when vetoing Pennsylvania's 1905 legislation, they noted that if they found the state's intervention legitimate in cases like Alice Smith's, "the doctrine we shall have enunciated cannot stop there."

There were other conditions besides epilepsy and the other enumerated statutory "defects" that might render persons a perceived burden to the common good. "Racial differences, for instance, might afford a basis for such (a policy) in communities where that question is unfortunately a permanent and paramount issue." Further, "Even beyond all such considerations it might be logically consistent to bring the philosophic theory of Malthus to bear upon the police power to the end that the tendency of population to outgrow its means of subsistence should be counteracted by surgical interference of the sort we are now considering." Having noted the logical destination of state intervention based on public health concerns and differential assessment of **social worth**, the New Jersey court decided not to decide this issue. Constitutional issues surrounding collective interests that might permit or even call for state intervention remained cloudy. The Supreme Court would clarify this issue in *Buck v. Bell* a decade and a half later.

There was, however, a less clouded constitutional issue. Equals should be treated equally. For cases like Alice Smith's it was clear "the force of the statute falls wholly upon such epileptics as are inmates confined in the several charitable institutions in the counties and State." If the public's health was accepted as a legitimate rationale and was to be protected by the elimination of procreation among epileptics and other "defectives" it would require "the sterilization of the vastly greater class who are not protected from procreation by their confinement in state or county institutions." If incarcerated epileptics were sterilized in the interest of the public's health, so should non-institutionalized epileptics. Failure to do so would undermine the entire policy.

For Alice Smith, the New Jersey Supreme Court found "the present statute is invalid in that it denies … the equal protection of the laws to which under the Constitution of the United States she is entitled." Judged to be inequitable, the law was no law at all. Alice Smith was not sterilized. The state could intrude in these extremely personal matters, but it had to do so equitably. In the years ahead similar issues came up in cases appealed in Michigan and New York, both decided in 1918.[3]

The New Jersey, Michigan, and New York cases also raised issues of equal protection. Other cases from other states involved the legitimacy of sterilization as punishment. Taken together these various concerns were addressed in Laughlin's 1922 model statute. While preparing his 1922 report, Laughlin had been working with Harry Olson, supervising judge for the Chicago Municipal Court. Judge Olson was also an active participant in the eugenics movement, at one time president of the Eugenics Research Association. Together, Olson and Laughlin decided that Laughlin's analysis and model statute should be widely distributed to politicians, judges, and activists across the country in an attempt to stimulate renewed interest in the faltering eugenic sterilization efforts (Laughlin 1922).

Laughlin's 1922 model statute provided a template for legislative change that would be widely debated.[4] Within two years of its release, some fifteen states passed laws patterned to greater and lesser degree after Laughlin's recommended language. Among these was Virginia's law, passed in 1924. It would soon move to the national forefront.

A Landmark Case Is Contrived

Reflecting the racial climate of the times as well as more specific eugenic interests, Virginia's dual-pronged 1924 legislation included the Racial Integrity Act and what came to be known as the Sterilization Act. Both eventually became landmarks in U.S. Constitutional Law.

The Racial Integrity Act, greatly influenced by the writings of Madison Grant, aimed to prevent the weakening of the white race by prohibiting inter-racial marriages. Some forty years later, it was challenged and overturned in *Loving v. Virginia* (1967). Shortly thereafter, *Loving* was cited in two companion cases, best known for honoring individual autonomy and firmly establishing the right to privacy—*Roe v. Wade* (1973) and *Doe v. Bolton* (1973). Virginia's Sterilization Act reached the Supreme Court much sooner. The Court's finding was quite the opposite when it came to justifying state intrusion into an individual's privacy and autonomy.

---

3 *Haynes v. Lapeer* Cir. Judge, 201 Mich. 138, 144-45, 166 N.W.938, 940-41 (1918); *Osborne v. Thomson*, 103, Misc. 23, 33-36, 169 N.Y.S. 638,643-45, aff'd; 185 App. Div. 902, 171 N.Y.S. 1094 (1918).

4 Charles Davenport, Laughlin's boss, was much less adamant about sterilization and more in favor of simple institutional segregation. He also felt that Laughlin's obsessive attention to sterilization was having negative political consequences.

To say the 1924 Virginia Racial Integrity and Sterilization acts reflected the climate of the times, both racial and eugenic, is not to say that both were easily passed into law as part of a tidal wave of public consensus. They were not. There was serious opposition to the Sterilization Act. Very specific individual interests and beliefs among a small group of influential politicians, lawyers, physicians, and administrators accounted for its eventual legislative success.

Thanks to the meticulous work of Paul Lombardo (1985), we know the details of how three long-time personal friends and close professional associates, Albert Priddy, Aubrey Strode, and Irving Whitehead, crafted a successful strategy not only for the passage of Virginia's sterilization statute, but also for its eventual affirmation in 1927 by the Supreme Court. Harry Laughlin, Harry Olson, Arthur Estabrook, and Henry Goddard were also in the mix. Justice Oliver Wendell Holmes, another prominent supporter of the eugenics movement, provided the sought after stamp of approval in *Buck v. Bell* (1927). By virtually any standard *Buck v. Bell* is a landmark case. It not only stands as a high-water mark for the eugenics movement, but also as a grounding reference point for when state intrusion overrides individual autonomy when no criminal wrong has been asserted or proven. The story took almost 15 years to unfold and begins about the time the ERO was getting off the ground in Cold Spring Harbor.

In 1910, Virginia, at the urgings of then State Senator Aubrey Strode, established the Virginia Colony for Epileptics and Feebleminded, eventually known simply as the Lynchburg Colony. It was located in Strode's home district and would become one of, if not the, largest such institution in the United States. Eventually, Virginia would become second only to California in the number of nonconsensual sterilizations performed.[5] The Colony's first three-member governing board included Irving P. Whitehead, Aubrey Strode, and Dr. Albert Priddy, the Colony's first superintendent.

In the 1916 session of the legislature, Senator Strode, working with Dr. Priddy, introduced five separate bills related to the treatment of the feebleminded. The most important of these proposals allowed sterilization without explicitly mentioning the procedure. Instead, the superintendent of the Colony and members of the Colony's Board were given authority to use moral, medical, and surgical treatments they deemed appropriate to promote the institution's mission. One of the institution's objectives was the protection of society.

Priddy's interpretation of the bill's language was clear. Within five days of the law's effective date, on June 9, 1916, he petitioned the Colony's Board for permission to sterilize eight women, using salpingectomy procedures. The three-member board responded in short order. With one member absent and one not responding,

---

5 For a documentary detailing sterilization in the Lynchburg Colony see *The Lynchburg Story: Eugenic Sterilization in America,* Stephen Trombley, 1994.

Whitehead alone provided written approval the same day Dr. Priddy's request was received. This quick turnaround soon became the rule. Requests to authorize sterilization and subsequent board approval were for the most part routine and perfunctory, with Priddy recommending and Whitehead approving, at times involving more than two dozen women in a single hearing.

Less than a year later, in March of 1917, the sterilization of two women, a mother and daughter, Miss Jessie Mallory and Mrs. Willie Mallory, was approved and the sterilizations were performed soon after. Two months later the father and husband filed three suits. Two were for the release of the younger Mallory children who had been taken into custody in the same raid on the family home, while the father was absent. These were successful and resulted in the release of the children. The third suit was for $5,000 in damages related to Mrs. Mallory's confinement and her subsequent forced sterilization.

In Mrs. Mallory's case, a jury returned a verdict in favor of Dr. Priddy. It was based on his defense that the sterilization had been performed for therapeutic reasons. Still, the judge was cautious and warned Priddy to discontinue his sterilization practices until the law could be clarified and strengthened. The judge was aware that depositions taken during the proceedings revealed serious questions about the legitimacy of the practices that resulted in Mrs. Mallory's commitment and sterilization. Dr. Priddy heeded the judge's concerns, but only in part. Sterilizations continued, but his stated rationale shifted. Instead of references to women of the "moron type," justifications for sterilizations were given, following the Mallory trial, in terms of relief of physical suffering for "pelvic disease" of unspecified origin.

While Priddy continued to claim he could treat his patients as he saw fit, he knew a new law was needed to provide adequate legal cover for his actions. Priddy provided a friend in the legislature with a draft bill, but this proposed legislation failed, garnering only a single vote, that of the bill's sponsor. In later correspondence a sympathetic physician colleague who had helped with the effort would note, "We were rewarded for our trouble by one vote and were laughed at by the law-makers" (Lombardo 1985: 45, fn 79).

There was support but there was also growing opposition from respected scientists who questioned the scientific validity of family pedigree studies and the claim that defects such as feeblemindedness were hereditary.[6] Such traits might run in the same family, but could be accounted for by any number of social, cultural, and economic explanations besides hereditary influence. In addition, the Catholic Church began

---

6   For example, in addition to the questions raised by anthropologists such as Franz Boas and Margaret Mead, Nobel Laureate, Hermann Joseph Muller, known for his work establishing a link between radiation and genetic mutation, had spoken out strongly against the implications of the family pedigree studies at the Third International Congress of Eugenics.

speaking in louder voice questioning the moral standing of mandatory sterilization. Despite this growing opposition, with the support of the General Board of State Hospitals, in 1923 Priddy and Strode again crafted legislation.

This time they used Laughlin's 1922 revised model sterilization statute as a touchstone for their proposed law. The bill, guided through the legislative process by Strode, reflected many of the details from Laughlin's template. It provided for "the sexual sterilization of inmates of state institutions in certain cases." The legislation passed both houses of Virginia's Assembly with only two dissenting votes. Still, there were worries whether the statute would withstand an appeal. Other laws had passed in other states only to be declared unconstitutional. Care should be taken.

Noting the importance of securing legitimacy through the appellate courts, the board directed Priddy to work with Strode to prepare a test case. They agreed. No sterilizations should take place before the new law was tested in the courts and placed on firm legal footing. The Lynchburg Colony needed a compelling, safe case to run through the courts. They also needed a strategy that would ensure success. They chose the case of an 18-year-old woman, Carrie Buck. In a clear conflict of interest, Irving Whitehead was asked to represent Carrie Buck. Aubrey Strode took the case on behalf of the state. Priddy, was the named defendant. It was a close-knit group. It would be a carefully coordinated effort. In the end, it was hard to argue that Carrie Buck's interests had been defended.

For the state, Strode wrote to Arthur Estabrook, who had been his wife's social work professor, asking him to assist in the evaluation of the Buck family. Two additional doctors, Albert Priddy and Joseph DeJarnette, were asked to testify. Priddy's self-interest in the case was evident. Dr. DeJarnette's was only a little less so. He had assisted Priddy in his failed legislative drafting, and had been the one complaining of legislative derision when their failed legislative attempt generated a single vote, accompanied by laughter in the legislature. Harry Laughlin, whom Priddy may have met during a visit to Judge Harry Olson's court a few years earlier and whom was certainly known by his leading role in the eugenics movement, was asked to provide a deposition as an expert witness. While he did not talk with Carrie Buck or any member of her family directly, Laughlin did receive correspondence from Priddy summarizing the case. He was quick to put it to use.

On the basis of this correspondence, Laughlin strongly supported the claim that Carrie Buck was a feebleminded and otherwise unfit individual whose traits were hereditary. In Laughlin's expert opinion, shaped by the letter he had received from Priddy, Carrie was a strong candidate for eugenic sterilization. With sometimes verbatim parroting of Priddy's words, Laughlin concluded, the Buck family belonged "... to the shiftless, ignorant, and worthless class of anti-social whites of the South ..."

In Carrie's defense, attorney Whitehead called no witnesses. Nor did he cross-examine or question in any detail witnesses or evidence provided by Strode. Carrie Buck had been chosen because of the assertion that her mother, she, and her daughter were all feeble-minded and that there was a family history of immoral, anti-social behavior. Whitehead could have challenged all of these assertions with substantial, easily available supporting evidence (Lombardo 1985: 50–55). He did not. It was by any standard a shoddy, feeble, and irresponsible defense.

The County Circuit Court affirmed the sterilization decision in February of 1925. Just a month prior to this decision, Dr. Priddy died and his assistant James H. Bell took over as the Colony's Superintendent, giving the case its new title, *Buck v. Bell*. Appeal was taken to the Virginia Supreme Court of Appeals, where the County Court's judgment was affirmed. Shortly after this decision, Strode and Whitehead jointly appeared before the Colony Board to celebrate their victory. Remembering that Strode and Whitehead were on opposite sides of the case, the notes of a subsequent meeting read in part, "... Colonel Aubrey E. Strode and Mr. I. P. Whitehead appeared before the Board ... their advice being that this particular case was in admirable shape to go to the court of last resort, and that we could not hope to have a more favorable situation than this one" (Lombardo 1985: 56). The assessment of the chances for success, by these clearly colluding lawyers, would prove correct.

The final step to firmly secure Virginia's Sterilization Act's constitutional legitimacy was the U.S. Supreme Court. Arguments were heard on April 22, 1927. A week and a half later, on May 2, Justice Oliver Wendell Holmes, on behalf of an 8–1 Court majority, issued the opinion affirming Virginia's sterilization statute (*Buck v. Bell* 1927). The Court found that Carrie Buck was a feeble-minded woman committed through appropriate procedures to the Virginia Colony for Epileptics and Feeble Minded. She was the daughter of a feeble-minded mother and the mother of an illegitimate, feeble-minded child. The decision to sterilize her had been reached through compliance with "very careful provisions" that protected patients from possible abuse. "So far as procedure is concerned," the Court concluded, "the rights of the patient are most carefully considered ... there is no doubt ..." Carrie Buck "... has had due process of law."

Turning from procedure to the issue of whether sterilization was ever appropriate as a eugenic public health measure, Justice Holmes grounded the opinion in the common good:

> We have seen more than once that the public welfare may call upon the best citizens for their lives. It would be strange if it could not call upon those who already sap the strength of the State for these lesser sacrifices ... in order to prevent our being swamped with incompetence ... The principle that sustains compulsory vaccination is broad enough to cover cutting the Fallopian tubes.

Closing with what reads like a frustrated comment from a member of the privileged class, Holmes wrote *Buck v. Bell*'s most famous sentence: "Three generations of imbeciles are enough." Perhaps never has such a strong condemning statement been written by such a respected jurist on the basis of such shoddy evidence. One can only speculate about whether it came in some measure from Holmes's personal and ardent support of the eugenics movement (Alschuler 2000: 27–30).

The final paragraph of the *Buck* decision addressed the issue of equal protection stemming from the fact that the statute did not apply to the feebleminded "multitudes outside." Holmes brushed this off as the "usual last resort of constitutional arguments." The law is never perfect, he noted. It "does all that is needed when it does all that it can." Case closed. Carrie Buck was sterilized five and a half months later on October 19, 1927.

The Floodgates Open

If ever there was a case that opened the floodgates, it was *Buck v. Bell*. Holmes's decision lay to rest issues of due process, equal protection and the legitimacy of mandated sterilization. In support of the decision, prominent theologians and legal scholars continued to assert, well into the 1950s, that the collective good could not be achieved "if the community may not defend itself, and is forced to permit the continued procreation of feeble-minded or hereditarily diseased children. Sterilization in such cases is not solely a matter of (personal control), but also of (state control)" (Fletcher 1954: 168).

State legislatures across the country took notice. According to data collected by the Human Betterment Foundation, by January 1933, 28 states had mandatory sterilization statutes. Starting the count in 1919, a total of just over 16,000 persons were nonvoluntarily sterilized—roughly 7,000 males and 9,000 females. In some states, e.g., California, the ratio of males to females was roughly 1 to 1. In states such as Kansas, males were at higher risk at a ratio of 1.5. In other states, the ratio was heavily weighted toward females. For example, in Minnesota approximately 10 females were sterilized for every male. By 1933, there had been a shift in these ratios toward more female sterilization when a new, simpler, and somewhat safer procedure, eventually known as the Pomery method of tubal ligation, was introduced to a wider audience in 1929 (Bishop and Nelms 1930: 214–16).

The states with the highest numbers mandatory sterilizations were spread from coast to coast, with California leading the way at 8,500, Virginia 1,300, Kansas and Michigan 1,000, Oregon 900, and Minnesota 700. There was a dramatic rise in mandated sterilizations in 1929 and another, even higher peak, roughly 5,000 nationwide, in 1932, the year prior to the passage of the initial German sterilization law. Subsequent yearly totals leveled off at roughly 3,000. This only slightly bumpy plateau held well into the 1940s (Reilly 1987: 162).

The isolated nature of institutions and a culture of professional independence among physicians, coupled with spotty record keeping across states and jurisdictions, means that precise totals and comparisons are suspect. All accounts, however, corroborate a dramatic increase in the number of nonconsensual sterilizations following *Buck v. Bell*, though even these are probably lower limit estimates.

Public Health Measures Go Terribly Wrong

Justice Holmes wrote in *Buck* it would be strange if the state "… could not call upon those who already sap the strength of the State for these lesser sacrifices … in order to prevent our being swamped with incompetence." In his opinion, as well as that of seven of his Supreme Court colleagues, the principle of supporting public health through mandatory sterilization was secure. In related, personal correspondence this same esteemed justice, son of the privileged, had also expressed his support for "putting to death the inadequate" and "infants that didn't pass the examination" (Alschuler 2000: 27–30). This was the kind of extended exclusionary logic that so troubled Governor Pennypacker and Judge Garrison. These principles of law were broad enough to justify far more extensive state intervention into the lives of individuals. Persons could be used, without their consent, for the good of the whole.

In the wake of *Buck*, mandated sterilizations in the United States increased. In subsequent years the evidence is now clear, there were also a series of medical experiments carried out using those on the margins of life to support the common good. Nothing, however, compared to what was about to happen in Germany. In July 1933, six months after Adolf Hitler became Chancellor, *Gesetz zur Verhütung Erbkranken Nachwuchses* (Law for the Prevention of Genetically Diseased Offspring) was enacted. The journey toward the Final Solution began.

This German statute, clearly an amalgam of Laughlin's 1922 template and more broadly drawn objectives, became effective on January 1, 1934. Following its passage, the next edition of the Eugenics Record Office's *Eugenics News*, where Harry Laughlin was a member of the editorial board, published a favorable review of the German statute, beginning by noting that Germany was the first of the world's major nations to enact a modern eugenical sterilization law for the nation as a whole.The parallels with their own work were noted with pride, as the German statute read almost like the American model sterilization law Laughlin had produced. In addition to Laughlin's model statute, Germany's newly formed government took note of Gosney and Popenoe's book, *Sterilization for Human Betterment*, and related work of the Human Betterment Foundation.

Traveling through Germany in 1934, an HBF board member reported to Gosney that their work was playing "… a powerful part in shaping the opinions of a group of intellectuals who are behind Hitler in this epoch-making program. Everywhere I sensed that their opinions have been tremendously stimulated by American thought, and particularly by the work of the Human Betterment Foundation" (Black 2002:

277).[7] A third element of American law and policy the Germans noted when passing the 1933 sterilization statute were the numerous statutes then on the books in the United States; statutes precipitated and legitimized by the U.S. Supreme Court's vindication of mandatory sterilization in *Buck v. Bell*.

The American roots of Germany's aggressive moves to limit "useless eaters" were further deepened through the financial support of the Rockefeller Foundation to the Kaiser Wilhelm Institute for Anthropology Human Heredity and Eugenics (founded in 1927) and the Kaiser Wilhelm Institute for Psychiatry. Located near the center of political power in Berlin and Munich and run by such academic and medical luminaries as Eugen Fischer, Fritz Lenz, Ernst Rüdin, and Otmar von Verschuer, these facilities became the leading force for eugenics in Germany. They would also eventually become closely tied to the sterilization of the so-called Rhineland Bastards, the infamous Aktion T4 program, and medical experiments conducted in Auschwitz (Weingart 1989).

The link between science and politics was crystal clear. A prominent German scientist and professor of medicine, Eugen Fischer, reporting on the activities of the KWI he was directing in Berlin, noted optimistically in 1941:

> The coming victorious end of the war and the monumental extension of the 'Greater German Empire' also present our research agencies with new tasks ... In times like these (we have) to serve the immediate interests of the people, the war, and politics; but second, (we) must orient (ourselves) to the future as well as the present, for one can never know what practical effects pure scientific research might have in the future ... No one could imagine that Gregor Mendel's studies of peas would provide the basis for a hereditary health legislation ... or that my study of bastards of 1908 could support race legislation. (Weingart 1989: 227)

There is now a well-documented story of how state imposed atrocities, grounded in the idea that society's defective outcasts, those seen as a burden to society, those referred to as "useless eaters," could be sterilized, experimented upon even to the point of disfigurement and death, for the good of the whole, began with the passage of Germany's encompassing sterilization law, explicitly patterned after Harry Laughlin's template. The underlying logic progressed step by step down a long and terrible road.

---

7 The full paragraph from the letter reads: "You will be interested to know that your work has played a powerful part in shaping the opinions of a group of intellectuals who are behind Hitler in this epoch-making program. Everywhere I sensed that their opinions have been tremendously stimulated by American thought, and particularly by the work of the Human Betterment Foundation. I want you, my dear friend, to carry this thought with you for the rest of your life, that you have really jolted into action a great government of 60,000,000 people."

These steps encountered political opposition along the way and required political campaigns to generate support. They took almost a decade to reach their final tragic climax (Lifton 1986; see also Alexander 1949: 39–47).

Ironically, each step included commitment to the idea that *LIFE* should be protected. Each step depended on exclusionary logic defining some lives as more worthy of protection, encouragement and support than others. In order to protect *LIFE*, some lives needed to be sacrificed. If respect for the dignity and autonomy of those less worthy had to be suspended, so be it.

This was the logic of the eugenics movement, eventually taken to the extreme, that so worried Governor Pennypacker, Judge Garrison and those who agreed with them. The debate and concerns would continue in the decades ahead. The revised understanding of the protective boundaries of life would be further informed by the not-well-understood implications of what came to be known as the biological revolution. Taken together, a moral and legal system was reshaped.

DISCUSSION QUESTIONS

1. Did you know much about the eugenics movement and its connection with what eventually became known as the Final Solution? If not, what questions now arise in your mind?
2. Did Priddy and Strode have adequate evidence that Carrie Buck was feeble-minded? If not, why do you think the Supreme Court upheld Virginia's law?
3. While most persons would reject the idea of mandatory sterilization for persons such as Carrie Buck, what are some of the other ways in which we develop a sense of differential social worth? What are the consequences of these assessments?

IV: Redrawing the Boundaries of Protected Life

＞＞＞×＜＜＜

Following World War II, the revelation of the Nazi atrocities, and the dropping of two atomic bombs, theologians, philosophers, physicians, lawyers, politicians, social scientists, and activists joined debate in a world where civil and human rights were being rethought, and where judgments regarding the protective boundaries of life were lagging behind advances in science and technology. General **Omar Bradley's** Armistice Day speech three short years after the annihilation of two Japanese cities is exemplary. Addressing his audience, Bradley warned:

> Our knowledge of science has clearly outstripped our capacity to control it ... Man is stumbling blindly through a spiritual darkness while toying with the precarious secrets of life and death. The world has achieved brilliance without wisdom, power without conscience. Ours is a world of nuclear giants and ethical infants....
>
> (1948)

General Bradley's assessment echoed across the social landscape. Moral and ethical frameworks were lagging dramatically behind scientific advances.

In pursuit of moral and ethical clarification, symposia were held, books written, social movements launched, academic and policy centers established, journals founded, governmental commissions convened, reports issued, regulations enacted, and Supreme Court decisions released. On all fronts, the goal was a clearer understanding of the boundaries of protected life, the meaning and importance of social worth, the dignity and respect accorded to autonomous individuals, and the allocation of authority to those who aimed to decide the fate of others.

Agreement was elusive. What was clarity and accurate assessment for some was obfuscation and flawed, even dangerous, thinking to others. Some six decades after World War II, in witness to the continuing uncertainties and contentious nature of the issues encountered, Leon Kass, a physician deeply concerned with the ethics of medical research would write, "The evils we face are intertwined with the goods we so keenly seek: cures for disease, relief of suffering, preservation of life. Distinguishing good and bad thus intermixed is often extremely difficult" (Kass 2002: 3).

An Awakening

There was one point, however, on which everyone agreed—German Nazis had engaged in barbaric behaviors. The stark nature of the suffering inflicted was jolting. The initial public response to the revealed Nazi atrocities, as intense as it was, was muted by a distancing collective denial. The quite specific roots the Nazi medical experiments shared with the eugenics movement advanced by Stanford University's first president, spearheaded by the director of the Eugenics Record Office at Cold Spring Harbor, legitimized by the Supreme Court, implemented in numerous sterilization statutes, and underwritten by the Rockefeller Foundation's contributions to the Kaiser Wilhelm Institutes in Germany and the T-4 unit and the Nazi euthanasia program ("The Rockefeller Foundation and the Kaiser Wilhelm Institute" 1936: 526–27), were rarely mentioned. German doctors and the system they defined were barbaric, but they were an anomaly. The war was over. The Allies had won. It was time to move on. There were, however, exceptions to this collective distancing and denial.

Shortly after World War II, a Boston physician focused his concerns about medical research more generally drawn in a widely influential article in the *New England Journal of Medicine* (Alexander 1949). Dr. Leo Alexander had been one of the architects of the Nuremberg Code used to prosecute German doctors ("Nuremberg Code" N.D.). He was worried. He knew the Nazi horrors had not sprung up instantly, but had been reached in small, incremental steps. He saw early danger signs among his medical colleagues in the United States:

> Whatever proportions these crimes finally assumed it became evident to all who investigated them that they had started from small beginnings. The beginnings at first were merely a subtle shift in emphasis in the basic attitude of the physicians. It started with the acceptance of the attitude, basic in the euthanasia movement, that there is such a thing as life not worthy to be lived.

In Dr. Alexander's mind, many of his colleagues had been similarly infected "with Hegelian, cold-blooded, utilitarian philosophy … early traces of it can be detected in their medical thinking that may make them vulnerable to departures of the type that occurred in Germany." (1949: 40) He wanted his readers to know if a patient could not be cured, physicians too often developed a sense of failure so that the "nonrehabilitable sick" too easily became "unwanted ballast." The impetus for Dr. Alexander's concerns was most importantly found in what some labeled **cultural lag** (Ogburn 1964).

Science, Technology, and Cultural Lag

The idea of cultural lag is straightforward. Science produces new knowledge. New knowledge is fashioned into innovative technologies. New technologies, especially those associated with the protection of life and the alleviation of suffering, call for moral and ethical refinements. The disjuncture between science, technology, and existing assessments of suffering and the protected boundaries of life is an important impetus for reshaping moral, legal, and ethical frameworks.

For persons such as Leo Alexander, the existing moral and legal frameworks were simply not up to the task. It was a well-recognized and increasingly discussed problem. Aldous Huxley in a reflective forward to his *Brave New World*, first published in 1932, reminded his readers, "The theme of the *Brave New World* is not the advancement of science as such; it is the advancement of science as it affects human individuals" (Huxley 1993: xi). Similarly, a pioneering practitioner in the use of artificial organs to sustain life, Dr. Belding Scribner, noted in his 1964 presidential address to the American Society for Artificial Internal Organs, "It is becoming increasingly clear that the moral and ethical guidelines handed down to us through the centuries are becoming more and more inadequate to govern our lives." Scribner urged his medical colleagues to join lawyers, theologians, and philosophers to "explore the possibility of some sort of joint effort in finding solutions to these vexing and urgent problems."

Given the uncertainty of shadowed legal and moral principles, as the debate moved forward disagreements emerged. Given the profound importance of the moral imperatives involved, these disagreements frequently become intense, and on occasion deadly.

A Crystallizing Event and Rationing Health Care

As is often the case, large questions and possible answers clarify in unexpected events. This became evident when Belding Scribner, working with engineering colleagues at the University of Washington in Seattle, developed a u-shaped arteriovenous cannula-shunt, made from the recently developed material, Teflon, and first used in 1960. This small device provided dramatically improved chances of surviving end-stage kidney disease. Patients confronting a 100 percent chance of near-term death now have access to multi-year survival.

In the beginning, the machines and procedures were limited, cumbersome and expensive. Who should be treated? Were some lives more worthy of saving than others? Who should decide? Answers to the ethical dilemmas and boundaries of relative worthiness embedded in these questions provided new impetus for how we rationed health care and thereby played an important role in the transformation the health care system (Jonsen 1990; Rothman 1991). After three patients had been successfully treated using the improved dialysis machine, University of Washington Hospital administrators informed Dr. Scribner that no new patients were to be accepted. The procedure was too expensive and the facilities too limited.

In short order the Seattle Artificial Kidney Center, connected with nearby Swedish Hospital, was established and opened for business in January 1962. It had three beds, associated dialysis equipment, and supporting medical personnel. Given the dramatic success of the new technology, demand for these new facilities immediately far exceeded what was available. Using the three beds, each patient would have to be hooked up for at least 10 hours, twice weekly. In the beginning it was decided that five patients could be served. Plans were put in place to expand this to 10. Difficult decisions would have to be made. Scribner, in his 1964 presidential address, noted that some 10,000 "ideal candidates" who could have been treated had died.

Two committees were set up. The Medical Advisory Committee, made up of physicians and a psychiatrist, would determine the initial pool of eligible patients. This screening would be based on emotional stability and medical prognosis. A second, the Admissions Advisory Committee, would determine who from this initial pool would be chosen. This seven-member committee included a lawyer, a housewife, an official of state government, a banker, a minister, a labor leader, and a surgeon. The membership was specifically designed to provide a non-medical assessment of the potential patients.

Random selection and first-come-first-served strategies were rejected. Decisions would be made on the basis of relative social worth. As stated, the role of the committee "was to assess the relative worth of a candidate to their family and the community in terms of the degree of dependence of others upon the candidate's continuing existence, and the rehabilitative potential and moral value or worth of the candidate" (Blagg 1998: 236). As impressive as the technological advances in dialysis were, it would be the necessity to ration health care guided by these vaguely specified criteria of relative worth that would capture the public's attention.

Shortly after the new dialysis center opened and the advisory committees convened, *Life* magazine, widely read for its pictorial spreads and accompanying journalistic accounts, sent a young west-coast staff writer, Shana Alexander, to Seattle to develop a story. It turned out to be the longest piece ever published by the magazine (Alexander 1962). Thirty years later, a conference was held in Seattle, bringing together 42 of the 60 individuals identified as bioethics pioneers, to commemorate Alexander's article as a crystallizing event in the launching of the bioethics movement (Jonsen 1993: S1). At the conference, Alexander characterized her story as the most "awesome and disturbing story" she had ever worked on (Alexander 1992).

Social Worth and Rationed Health Care

Alexander's story presented an early glimpse of how the uncertain assessment of life's potential and social worth would dominate moral debates in the years ahead. In one sense it was *déjà vu* as it raised the same question as the eugenics movement. Instead of regulating the ability to have children and thereby protect the health of the broader community, social worth was used to allocate life-prolonging resources. Increasingly effective immunosuppressant drugs and successful organ transplants were being developed, as were methods to maintain the lives of infants and adults who would have died in previous years. The questions were not likely to go away any time soon.

Beyond rough and ready rationing guidelines, there was little clarity. After briefing the Admissions Committee, a doctor recalled, "We told them frankly that there were *no* guidelines, they were on their own. We really dumped it on them." (This and quotes to follow are taken from Alexander 1962.) Committee members wanted to maximize their objectivity and therefore blocked knowledge of the attending physician and the name of the patient from their deliberations. If personal knowledge entered in, they would excuse themselves from the decision. Piece by piece, a template for assessing differential social worth and the boundaries of protected life began to take shape. It was a work in progress.

Ambiguities in judgments of relative worth as well as refinements in the committee's thinking became evident as their deliberations proceeded. Details were reconstructed in Alexander's article:

MINISTER: How can we compare a family situation of two children, such as this woman in Walla Walla, with a family of six children, such as patient Number Four—the aircraft worker?

STATE OFFICIAL: But are we sure the aircraft worker can be rehabilitated? I note he is already too ill to work, whereas Number Two and Number Five, the chemist and the accountant, are both still able to keep going.

LABOR LEADER: I know from experience that the aircraft company where this man works will do everything possible to rehabilitate a handicapped employee....

HOUSEWIFE: If we are still looking for the men with the highest potential for service to society, then I think we must consider that the chemist and the accountant have the finest educational backgrounds of all five candidates.

SURGEON: How do the rest of you feel about Number Three—the small businessman with three children? I am impressed that his doctor took special pains to mention that this man is active in church work. This is an indication to me of character and moral strength.

HOUSEWIFE: Which certainly would help him conform to the demands of the treatment....

LAWYER: It would also help him to endure a lingering death....

Uncertainty was unavoidable. As the lawyer on the committee noted in an interview with Shana Alexander, "I believe that a man's contribution to society should determine our ultimate decision. But I'm not so doggone sure that a great painting or a symphony would loom larger in my own mind than the needs of a woman with six children."

Committee members were also aware that implications of their criteria would soon expand. Successful organ transplants were just around the corner. As the surgeon on the Admissions Committee noted,

> Medically speaking, I am not a disciple of this particular approach to kidney disease. But in the larger view, this project will not just benefit one disease – it will benefit all aspects of medicine. We are hoping someday to learn how to transplant live organs. So far, the body will not accept foreign tissue from another person, but eventually we will find a way to break this tissue barrier.

The surgeon had reason to be optimistic. In the mid- to late 1950s and early 1960s work on kidney transplants was proceeding. In 1963, one year after the surgeon's interview, a spate of articles appeared in medical journals signaling promising success in the use of immunosuppressant drugs and related kidney transplant therapies (Hume et al. 1963; Murray et al. 1962, 1963; Starzl, Marchioro, and Waddell 1963; Woodruff et al. 1963). At the same time, demand was driving an increase in supply of kidney dialysis machines. By 1965 an estimated 800 persons were on **hemodialysis** in some 121 centers spread across the country. Even with this impressive expansion, the demand continued to far outdistance available resources. Estimates put the number of persons in need of hemodialysis between 60,000 and 90,000, with an increased number of between 5,000 and 10,000 each year (Sanders and Dukeminier 1968: 366). Patient selection and the rationing of access could not be avoided. It continued to be driven by assessments of social worth. For many, this was disturbing and offensive.

A sharp articulation of these objections came from a Director of Community Services at Cedars-Sinai Medical Center and his colleague, a Professor of Law at UCLA (Sanders and Durkheminier 1968). In their introduction, they wrote:

> The spectacular recent advances of medical science have created unprecedented legal and ethical problems ... Medical science is creating and allocating resources of the greatest value; use of the resource means life, denial means death ... If society, with its chief instrument, law, does not tame technology, technology may destroy our sense of ethics—and man himself.

Their critique was harsh. They characterized the Seattle Admissions Committee's decision framework as "a grotesque conceit worthy of Franz Kafka." In practice, the committee was doing nothing other than "measuring persons in accordance with its own middle-class suburban value system." It was simply the "bourgeoisie sparing the bourgeoisie." Creative, contributing nonconformists need not apply. "The Pacific Northwest," the authors wrote, "is no place for a Henry David Thoreau with bad kidneys" (413).

Pandora's box had been opened, and the issues were unavoidable. With the expansion of hemodialysis and organ transplant programs, the debate widened. If not social worth, then what? How should the boundaries protecting one life above another be drawn? If all lives are of equal value, why not set up a random selection procedure? Why not operate on a first-come-first-served basis? Why not let market forces determine access and simply save those who can pay? While each of these options presented problems, the authors of the *UCLA Law Review* piece concluded, "Any of these methods is preferable to selection by ad hoc comparative judgments of social worth." Many others disagreed with this conclusion. The debate would endure.

Stories are Told, Doctrines Explored

As physicians, philosophers, lawyers, and theologians struggled to clarify rationing standards for dialysis and organ transplants, they took notice of a *Harvard Law Review* article, written some 15 years earlier by Lon Fuller. In his 1949 article, Fuller told a story to make his point. It involved trapped spelunkers, who, after rolling dice, chose a companion to kill and eat in order to survive. The surviving spelunkers were tried, convicted of murder, and sentenced to hang. They appealed their case. Through the opinions of the appellate judges, Fuller explored various moral and legal issues related to the protection and termination of life under such dire circumstances. In the end, the conviction was affirmed and the defendants hanged.

This contrived account, while dramatic and based in general outline on actual and well-known cases, was of limited use as metaphor for choosing hemodialysis and organ transplant patients. The writings of another lawyer-philosopher, Edmond Cahn, also drew attention. The same year as Fuller's spelunker article appeared, Cahn had published *The Sense of Injustice*. While clearly relevant to the choice of patients for dialysis and organ transplants, Cahn's ideas were developed in a time when such choices were rarely contemplated let alone immediately present as unavoidable necessities. How did they apply to rationing health care? Not clear, was the answer.

Some additional clarity was found in Cahn's second book, *The Moral Decision*, published seven years before the Seattle hemodialysis clinic was established. In one section, "The Value of Being Alive," Cahn explored the actual cases underpinning Fuller's contrived spelunkers. One case involved an overloaded longboat cast adrift in freezing seas when the mother ship struck an iceberg. Decisions of who should be cast overboard were made by the first mate. When the survivors returned to Philadelphia there was talk of prosecution. All but the first mate disappeared. He was put on trial, convicted and sentenced to six months of hard labor in addition to the nine months he had spent in jail awaiting trial.

What lessons could be learned from these experiences? For Cahn, every human life has some value but under some circumstances, some may be more worthy than others.

How to decide? Given the continuing elusiveness of the criteria for determining differential social worth, and viewing all life as valuable, Cahn turned to the virtue of volunteers. Let the virtue of those most immediately involved determine the outcome. In the longboat, virtue was rare and volunteers few. Selfish interests dominated. Most male passengers did not volunteer to lighten the boat. Instead, they had tried by offers of bribes and the use of force to stay aboard. Lacking virtuous volunteers and acceptable criteria for assessing social worth, reliance on the invisible hand of destiny became ever more attractive.

Taking action to kill some so that others might live was not acceptable to Cahn. Absent volunteers and clear criteria for choosing, Cahn was personally drawn to letting destiny determine the outcome. For Cahn, intentionally killing, even in these extreme circumstances, was not acceptable. As interesting as Cahn's analysis was, those looking for guidelines to ration hemodialysis and organ transplants found little guidance.

With transplants and dialysis, the choice, no matter if by casting lots or social worth, was not who should be killed first, but who should first be rescued. Doing good, knowing harm would result was a pervasive and long-contemplated dilemma. Theologians had struggled with the issue for centuries, developing in the process the **Doctrine of Double Effect**. As debates progressed, this doctrine received increased interest. In particular Philippa Foot, a philosopher introduced in 1967 what came to be known as the **Trolley Problem** (Foot 1967). The Trolley Problem took numerous forms. Whatever the specifics, it always presented a forced choice of doing good, knowing bad would result. The trolley problem and related metaphors, illustrating the double effect of intended and **unintended consequences**, would arise repeatedly in the years ahead (see, for example, Thomson 1971, 1976; and Woodard 2001). By the late 1960s, broad guidelines were beginning to take shape.

The Decade of Conferences

The utility of general concepts such as "social worth," "intention," and "double effect" are that they shed common light on otherwise diverse situations such as eugenics, abortion, neonatal care, patient choice, and both active and passive euthanasia. When applied to particular situations, however, specification is always necessary.

These general concepts and specific implications were repeated explored in what has been labeled the "Decade of Conferences" (Jonsen 1998: 13; Jonsen's book remains the most comprehensive account of the emergent bioethics movement). In the 1960s, doctors, philosophers, theologians, social scientists, lawyers, and political activists wrote papers, published books, convened symposia, identified criteria, crafted principles, and drafted laws to frame the meaning of what came to be known as bioethics: a framework that would provide useful guideposts for finding our way through "the rapid and awesome advances of contemporary science in controlling the physical and mental processes of human life (Labby 1966).

Some of these conferences, such as the Dartmouth Convocation on Great Issues of Conscience in Modern Medicine in 1960 (*Dartmouth Alumni Magazine* 1960), and the *Sanctity of Life* symposium, held at Reed College in 1966, asked sweeping questions such as: "Could one identify the forces in society that determine how valuable one man holds the life of another? Do adequate guidelines exist in law, theology, or in the liberal arts? Are the biomedical sciences, dedicated to preserving health and prolonging life, taking undue liberties in the guise of improving man's condition?" (Labby 1966: ix). Within these broad questions, conference participants tackled topics ranging from eugenics and the creation of sperm banks to global issues of environmental degradation, nuclear war, and how the elimination of certain diseases might impact population growth among the world's most impoverished people.

Other symposia were more narrowly organized around particular issues. Proceedings from one such conference, drawing participants from eight countries, were published in 1966 as *Ethics in Medical Progress: With special reference to transplantation*. One reviewer of the conference would note, "This book might well have been subtitled 'What Price My Kidney?'" (Harvey 1967).

Broadly drawn or narrowly focused these gatherings brought together a stellar array of the academic and professional elite.[1] With the exception of abortion and concerns for the environment, broad-based political action groups had yet to assert themselves. Instead, the public was "seen as an audience, waiting for scientists to bring solutions to the problems they have created" (Jonsen 1963: 15). Conferences were informed by the now well-known double-helix structure of DNA. Several other highly promising advances, limiting the spread of disease and providing life-saving technologies, such as hemodialysis, organ transplantation, and respirators drew substantial attention. Conference participants grappled repeatedly with forced-choice dilemmas of who should live and who should die, reflecting an awakened awareness that scientific knowledge and all good intentions might go terribly wrong. Innovations benefiting some could and did have negative even devastating implications for others.

Flawed Judgment and Sloppy Science

Some negative consequences of scientific advances came directly from flawed judgment and sloppy science. Addressing these issues during the 1966 Reed College *Sanctity of Life* conference, Dr. Henry K. Beecher noted, "One often hears it said these days

---

1 For one listing of many of the prominent players focusing on medical aspects of these issues see Jonsen 1993: S 16.

that moral choices are always among shades of gray, never between black and white. This, of course, is not true" (1968: 116).

What most concerned Beecher were experiments using humans without their consent. This was a black and white issue. It should not be done. Beecher had set the stage for his damning conference critique in an article in the *Journal of the American Medical Association* in 1959. His conference talk was largely an update of this article as well as a reprise and elaboration of his more recently published piece in the *New England Journal of Medicine*, which would help precipitate medical research reforms in the years just ahead (Beecher 1999).

Dr. Beecher had personal experience to draw upon. He was an endowed faculty member at Harvard Medical School, and, while controversial, he was generally considered among the world's foremost anesthesiologists. He was well versed in the Nazi human experiments, which had led to the trial of 23 doctors, 7 of whom had been executed and 9 others sent to prison. He knew well that the Nuremberg Code began with the sentence: "The voluntary consent of the human subject is absolutely essential."

Like Leo Alexander, Henry Beecher also knew that violations of this principle, as well as principles embedded in the Declaration of Helsinki, adopted by the 18th World Medical Assembly held in Helsinki, Finland, in June of 1964 were not restricted to the horrors of Nazi medical experiments. They were present in research being done in reputable hospitals and universities across the United States and in the clandestine experiments conducted by the CIA on mind-altering drugs and mind-control techniques. The military was doing research involving human subjects to better understand radiation effects associated with the fallout from atomic bomb use and testing (see McCoy 1966; Welsome 1999). Beecher knew and acknowledged also that even some of his own practices were not above reproach. Leo Alexander's earlier warning that Americans should be aware that Nuremberg Code violations were present in their own midst was clear.

With this background and the knowledge that his colleagues attending the Reed College conference in Oregon would be uncomfortable with his message, Dr. Beecher set out to document his concerns. The problem was, Beecher told his audience, the focus of clinical research was not on healing the patient. It was investigating the disease. Persons were being used to achieve a "greater good." There were clear dangers in such investigations. As serious as these dangers already were, Beecher went on, they were likely to increase in the coming years due to increased federal funding, the promise of new knowledge, and academic pressure on investigators to produce results.

From 22 studies, culled from the 50 he had been looking into, Beecher noted evidence clearly documenting that hundreds of patients had not known they were subjects of experiments, though grave harm had been suffered. While some might argue that the greater good justified this suffering, Beecher was not among them. Science was not the highest value to which all other orders and values should be subordinated.

The real problem for Beecher, however, was not intentional harm. Instead, during the ten years of his study of these matters it had become apparent that thoughtlessness and carelessness had led physicians and researchers to risk the health or the life of their subjects. Beecher's argument was compelling. Later evidence only confirmed his assertions (see, Oral History of the Belmont Report and the National Commission for the Protection of Human Subjects of Biomedical and Behavioral Research, 2004: 5; Pappworth 1962). Tighter controls to minimize carelessness were needed. The need would become glaringly clear in the early 1970s when three highly questionable, decades-long studies, including one Beecher had noted, came to the public's attention. All three studies involved underprivileged patients at the social and economic margins of life, patients whose lives were deemed less worthy of careful protective safeguards than others.

When Dr. Henry Beecher was speaking in Oregon and publishing in the *New England Journal of Medicine*, publicity surrounding these troubling events was yet to come, but reforms were in the works (Memorandum 1966). First, however, there was another matter in need of immediate attention. Once again, dramatic scientific and technological breakthroughs called for rethinking the protective boundaries of life.

Harvesting for Life

Concerns with the ethics of using human subjects in clinical studies had led Harvard to establish a Standing Committee on Human Studies, with Dr. Beecher as its chair. Dr. Joseph Murray, who was later awarded the Nobel Prize in Medicine for his work on kidney transplants, was one of Beecher's colleagues. Both were aware of unresolved ethical issues raised by rapidly improving organ transplant procedures and the increasing effectiveness of immunosuppressant drugs. They were also convinced these issues, like the ethics of medical research involving humans, would become increasingly pressing. There was an immediate need of clarification.

Long-established common law definitions of death were no longer as useful as they once were. They relied on the absence of cardio-respiratory activity. Readily available technology now meant respiration and blood circulation could be artificially maintained for years in some cases. Waiting too long to harvest organs meant they would deteriorate. Harvesting too soon presented obvious ethical and legal issues. Defining death in terms too closely tied to probabilities of successful transplantation presented vexing problems too obvious to ignore. The outdated definition of death made so evident by new technologies demanded attention.

These issues came to a head when late in the evening of December 3, 1967, in Cape Town, South Africa, Dr. Christiaan Bernard transplanted a heart taken from a young woman in her early twenties, Denise Ann Darvall. Denise had been critically injured in a car accident earlier that morning, suffering a skull fracture and serious brain injuries. She could not be kept alive without "artificial" means.

Around 9:00 that evening her heart and kidneys were removed with the permission of her father.

Her kidneys were given to 10-year-old Jonathan van Wyk, a "coloured" boy, which caused some short-lived controversy in apartheid South Africa since Denise was white. The recipient of her heart was a 55-year-old grocer, Louis Washkansky. Dr. Barnard's operation drew world-wide attention, and while Mr. Washkansky survived less than three weeks, he was seen as the recipient of the first successful human heart transplant. Given the circumstances surrounding Denise Durvall's organ removal and transplantations, the pressing nature of broader ethical questions loomed large. More such operations were sure to come. A clearer example of cultural lag could not be imagined.

Two months prior to when Denise Ann Darvall's heart was transplanted into the body of Louis Washkansky, Dr. Beecher had written the dean of the Harvard Medical School suggesting that the Human Studies Committee's charge be expanded. His rationale was clear. "Both Dr. Murray and I think the time has come for a further consideration of the definition of death. Every major hospital has patients stacked up waiting for suitable donors" (cited in Rothman 1991: 160–61). Shortly after Washkansky's death on December 21, 1967, the Dean of Harvard Medical School, on January 4, 1968, heeded Beecher and Murray's request and established what came to be known as the Harvard Brain Death Committee. Henry Beecher would be its chair. Physicians dominated the committee, but additional members were chosen for their expertise in theology, history, law, and ethics. These same issues were drawing attention in Washington D.C..

Deference to Doctors

Concern for the ethics of medical research, along with the drama of the first human heart transplants[2] and other rapidly advancing medical technologies and procedures, had captured the attention of some in the U.S. Senate. Prominent among them was Senator Walter Mondale. In 1968, a month after the Harvard committee began its work, Senator Mondale introduced legislation to establish a Presidential Study Commission on Health Science and Society. Hearings were held in March and April as Mondale called upon a parade of prominent physicians and scientists, both for and against establishing such a commission. These included Henry Beecher, speaking in favor of establishing the Study Commission, and Christiaan Bernard, who drew a packed hearing room when he testified in strong opposition.

Beecher reaffirmed his belief that there were limits beyond which medical science, even in search of life enhancing remedies, should not pass. These needed to be better

---

2 Denton Cooley, operating in Houston Texas, performed a second human heart transplant in June this same year.

defined and a Study Commission would be useful. Theologian Kenneth Vaux agreed, and with biblical allusion to the consequences of passing these limits, noted, "what will it profit us if we gain the whole world and forfeit our soul?" (cited in Jonsen 1993: 92). The argument from those in opposition was that government commissions were cumbersome and would produce needless, counterproductive regulations. As the now celebrated heart surgeon, Dr. Barnard, put it, "I do not think the public is qualified to make the decision…. You must leave it in the people's hands who are capable of doing it" (cited in Rothman 1991: 172–73). Christiaan Barnard's argument would carry the day. The 1968 hearings closed without producing legislation. Trust in those "capable of doing it," for the time being, remained secure. This would soon change.

A Paradigm for Protected Life

The stage for what came to be known as the bioethics movement was firmly set in 1969 when theologian James Gustafson organized a final gathering of the decade, cosponsored by Yale Divinity School, where Gustafson taught, and the Yale School of Medicine. The conference would prove to be highly influential.

Gustafson was a well-respected scholar and had recently written about the numerous conferences being held. "One hopes we can move beyond the conference procedure," Gustafson wrote, "to a more disciplined, careful, long range way of working in which areas of disagreement can not only be defined but in part at least overcome." What was needed, he concluded, was the mobilization and organization of resources, "interdisciplinary work within universities or centers that have personnel and resources for the arduous tasks of intensive and long-term work" (Gustafson 1968: 27–30).

Gustafson organized the gathering with these objectives in mind. Its featured speaker, around whom the proceedings were organized, was Paul Ramsey. It would later be written that this "massive" conference was enlivened by vigorous panel responses to Ramsey's presentations and "marked the beginnings of a new and astoundingly influential scholarly practical discipline" (Farley 2002).

Ramsey was a widely recognized, outspoken Christian ethicist from Princeton, known as an acute analytic scholar and a sometimes acerbic, argumentative, and strong-willed talker. At previous conferences he had repeatedly challenged the "shallowness of scientists' moral thinking about abortion and genetics." He did so again, though this time his criticisms would be broader based and more fully developed.

Having received the first grant given by the Joseph P. Kennedy Jr. Foundation for studying medical ethics, Ramsey took the unusual step of preparing for his presentations by spending the better part the spring semesters in 1968 and 1969 talking with and observing doctors and scientists at Georgetown University School of Medicine. Drawing on this experience and his background as a theologian and ethicist, he organized his presentations into four lectures: "Updating Death," "Caring for the

Dying," "Giving and Taking Organs for Transplantation," and "Consent in Medical Experimentation."

Thanking various participants attending the Yale conference, with wry, self-deprecating humor, Ramsey recalled, when delivering the first of his lectures, the words of a wise colleague:

> I should say that these lectures will ask more questions than they will answer, will pose questions that may be unanswerable, will answer questions seldom asked and particularly questions physicians never thought of asking, and won't answer the questions doctors did ask.
>
> I stipulate that to do any one of these things shall be deemed success and that I enroll in any of these undertakings only on a "Pass-Fail" basis. Stiffer competition or any more severe judgment would be too much for me.

Those in attendance, mostly northeastern physicians and Ivy League academics, may have smiled at these disarming introductory comments from a colleague they knew to be strong-willed and self-assured. Their smiles would soon fade. They recognized a scholarly tour de force when they saw one. As an extension and elaboration of his lectures, a year after the conference, Yale University Press published Ramsey's *The Patient as Person.*

Together, Ramsey's lectures and book extended and enriched the human rights principles embedded in the hastily crafted Nuremberg Code. They provided further grounding for the worried musings of Leo Alexander and Henry Beecher. They specified and humanized the philosophic generalizations regarding the importance of intentions and the Doctrine of Double Effect. With his lectures completed and *The Patient as Person* published, Ramsey's work became, without question, a cornerstone for the agenda of a field for which a term was about to be coined. They might "rightly be called the founding preaching and scriptures of the field of bioethics" (Jonsen 2002: xvi–xxvii).

DISCUSSION QUESTIONS

1. Cultural Lag is an enduring problem and an impetus for the evolution of moral systems. What are some additional examples to the ones provided in this chapter?
2. In what ways are the issues at the heart of allocating access to scarce medical resources related to the eugenics movement?
3. Should the government regulate the ethics of medical research, or should it be left in the hand of the physicians? Why?

V: Crystallizing Events and Ethical Principles

❧❧❧

With the intellectual stage set, the 1970s ushered in what might be called the Decade of Crystallizing Events. These events focused attention, clarified issues, galvanized effort, and precipitated a call for legislatively defined moral principles. The human tragedies embedded in these events energized legal reform efforts more effectively than conference presentations ever could.

A Term is Coined

Conference discussions throughout the 1960s encouraged a growing number of publications that covered the protective boundaries of life and tolerable suffering in the broadest sense (see, for example, Carmody 1970; Hall and Swenson 1968). But perspectives from the humanities, social, behavioral, and natural sciences, engineering, and medicine needed to be joined. An early proposal came from an oncologist working at the medical school at the University of Wisconsin in Madison.

Professor Van Rensselaer Potter was interested in the links between health and environmental carcinogens. Margaret Mead, the anthropologist, had inspired him with her calls for interdisciplinary study where the very survival of the human race and possibly of all living creatures depended upon a vision of the future for others, which commanded our deepest commitment. Potter had written various articles on related topics throughout the 1960s. In 1971, he brought some of his ideas together in *Bioethics: Bridge to the Future*, wherein he hoped to contribute to the future of the human species by promoting the formation of a new discipline. By most accounts, this small volume marked the coining of the term, bioethics.[1]

---

1 There is some academic debate over just who coined the term "bioethics." See Reich's companion articles: "The Word 'Bioethics': Its Birth and the Legacies of Those Who Shaped Its Meaning," 1994, and "The Word 'Bioethics': The Struggle over Its Earliest Meanings," 1995.

Two Centers Frame the Debate

While Potter was publishing his papers and coining a term, two research and teaching centers were being organized and the loosely knit Society of Health and Human Values (see McElhinney and Pelligrino 2001) was being founded by those who had been most involved in the conferences of the 1960s. The Hastings Center, located on the Hudson River a little over an hour drive from New York City, and the Kennedy Institute of Ethics (originally called the Joseph and Rose Kennedy Institute for the Study of Human Reproduction and Bioethics), at Georgetown University, in Washington D.C. eventually became the dominant framers of what came to be known as the bioethics movement.

The Hastings Center, by design, aimed to carve out a new field of scholarly discourse. Articles appearing in *The Hastings Center Report* (HCR) would shape much of the scholarly discussion in the years ahead as the Hastings Center became in many ways a "Leader of Leaders" (Stevens 2000). The Kennedy Institute's strategic location in the nation's capital, along with its ability to mobilize resources and organize effort, would be called upon repeatedly in support of numerous governmental commissions and landmark legal cases.

High on the early agenda for both the Kennedy Institute and the Hastings Center was what bioethics, as an interdisciplinary enterprise, should look like. Little emphasis was placed upon the abstract formulations of logicians and analytic philosophers; more upon practical concerns physicians, patients, and medical researchers. As Daniel Callahan, the first director of the Hastings Center, put it, the aim was to develop a discipline "so designed, and its practitioners so trained, that it will directly—at whatever cost to disciplinary elegance—serve those physicians and biologists whose position demands that they make the practical decisions" (1973:1). Fledgling bioethicists were drawn to the practical issues embedded in several high-profile events that came to light in the early 1970s. These events reinvigorated Senator Mondale's failed 1968 congressional hearings and calls for action. Drawn to these matters and encouraged by the stated purposes of their primary benefactor, members of the newly established Kennedy Institute responded and launched an "applied" endeavor aimed in large measure at ethical questions of medical research and practice.

Trust and singular reliance on the common sense of physicians who, as Christiaan Barnard had put it in testimony before Senator Mondale's 1968 Committee, were "capable of doing it" began to break down. Greater weight was given to the wisdom of those likeminded to Governor Pennypacker of Pennsylvania, who decades earlier when vetoing mandatory sterilization legislation, had stated, "(Physicians) of high scientific attainment are prone, in their love for technique, to lose sight of broad principles outside of their own domain of thought." Other perspectives were needed and oversight was called for. Congress would soon ask for both. As one observer noted,

"The formal birth of bioethics really began by Congressional mandate!" (Irving 2000: 1) This mandate was precipitated by four separate and disturbing accounts of highly questionable medical practices.

Four Crystallizing Events

In 1971, Senator Mondale, along with 17 congressional co-sponsors, reintroduced his 1968 proposal for a commission for the "study and evaluation of the ethical, social, and legal implications of advances in biomedical research and technology." As one of the founding members of the Hastings Center, Mondale's proposal to Congress was published in the first edition of *The Hastings Center Report*, "The Issues Before Us."

It was accompanied by a short inset, written by Paul Ramsey, urging the medical profession, scientists, and legislators, to give these issues the serious attention they deserved. It was too easy, Ramsey warned, "to raise ethical questions with a frivolous conscience and to no serious purpose." For Ramsey serious purpose meant that lawmakers, physicians, and scientists needed to be prepared to "stop the trial or procedure in question in the event that the 'ethical finding' should turn out to be murder or deception or other serious wrong to actual or (now) hypothetical human beings."

Senator Mondale's renewed call for legislative action initially gained little traction, passing the Senate, but failing to gather much attention in the House. Revelations of disturbing, issue-clarifying events calling for serious focused action changed this.

Just months after Senator Mondale presented his proposal, the *Washington Post*, on October 8, 1971, carried a front-page story with the headline, "Pentagon Has Contract to Test Radiation Effect on Humans." The lead paragraph stated:

> For the past 11 years, the Pentagon has had a contract with the University of Cincinnati to study the effects of atomic radiation on human beings. The prime purpose of the study, according to the contract, has been to "understand better the influence of radiation on combat effectiveness.

The head of the Cincinnati research team, Dr. Eugene Saenger, was quoted reaffirming his belief in the legitimacy and value of the project. "There is a need to investigate the effects of radiation on human beings to give support to the military ... These are tough problems that should not be swept under the rug, and I personally think the work we are doing is damned important."

The patients receiving radiation all had cancer. They were poor, with little education, unable to pay for private physicians. Just over 60 percent were of African-American heritage. All came to the hospital seeking help. There was little or no hope that the full-body radiation treatment would help them personally, but researchers believed that by monitoring such radiation effects they would learn something valuable to assist military personnel on the battlefield or citizens in the event of an atomic attack. In the minds of many, in a time of Mutually Assured Destruction (MAD), the potential knowledge gained was "damned important." The full extent to which similar radiation experiments were being conducted across the country during the Cold War would not come to light until years later (see, Little, Jr. 1972; J. Stephens 1973; M. Stephens 2002; Welsome 1999).

One thing, however, was immediately clear. There were strong parallels between the Cincinnati research and the practices and rationale German doctors had for conducting medical experiments during WWII. In Cincinnati, as in Germany, experiments were designed to shed light on how to protect the military under life-threatening conditions. In both instances, medical research, known to create painful and even lethal effects, was designed to advance knowledge, not improve the health of patients being treated. Both experiments were carried out without fully informed consent of the persons being studied. In both instances, the privileged and well-situated members of society were nowhere to be found among those being studied. In Cincinnati, as in Germany, one could easily detect the implied dehumanizing question: If patients of less social worth are going to die anyway, why not use them for the greater good? Had not just such a rationale been used by Justice Holmes in *Buck v. Bell* (1927) to justify mandatory sterilization?

The *Washington Post* revelation of the Cincinnati radiation experiments did not create instant and widespread outrage. It did, however, capture the attention of a few legislators and a young assistant professor of English, Martha Stephens, along with some of her colleagues in the Junior Faculty Association (JFA) at the University of Cincinnati. As a young faculty member, Stephens took it upon herself to approach the director of the university's medical center to get further details. It took some convincing. There was resistance to releasing the material and paternalistic comments from the physicians suggesting English professors might not understand the technical details. After several persistent visits, however, one afternoon Stephens walked into the director's office and saw a large stack of documents on the director's desk. "Here they are, if you really want them," he told her. She walked out of the office with "about six hundred pages of double-spaced transcript in several dark brown folders." Over the holidays she would read this material and write a report to her colleagues on the JFA.

It was a sobering experience. She read profiles doctors had appended to their annual reports, "I could readily see … that one patient had died six days after radiation, and others on day seven, day nine, day ten, fifteen, twenty, twenty-two, and so on." "It was clear" she concluded, "that these tests would have to be brought to an end and that any of us on campus who could help must do so." With her reading and research completed, on January 25, 1972, just under four months after the initial story broke, Stephens' seven-page report, addressed to "the campus community," was released in a press conference held by the JFA.

One person attending the press conference was a reporter from the *Washington Post*. He took the report and wrote a story that appeared the next day (Auerbach 1971: A3). At this same time, Senator Edward Kennedy was working with Senator Mondale and others to revive congressional interest in more effective regulation of medical experiments involving humans. Kennedy saw the *Post* story and read the JFA's conclusions into the Congressional Record. Following the press conference, Kennedy asked one of his aides to begin working with Professor Stephens and her colleagues. The medical community was challenging the JFA report and Kennedy wanted to find out more. Within two months, Senator Kennedy and Ohio Governor John Gilligan met with University of Cincinnati's president, Warren Bennis, and reached agreement to stop the research in question.

Momentum for reform involving tighter controls of medical research was building. It was further energized by three additional revelations. The first came from Staten Island the same month Martha Stephens and her colleagues released their JFA report. Again, there were charges of serious wrong being done to persons on the margins of protected life.

In his 1966 *New England Journal of Medicine* article, Henry Beecher had pointed to a research project that had taken place in an institution for mentally retarded children. He had not identified the institution, but the study was described as being directed "toward determining the period of infectivity of infectious hepatitis." It involved the "artificial induction of hepatitis … in an institution of mentally defective children in which a mild form of hepatitis was endemic."

As more specifically described in a later account, "The experiments typically involved injecting some of the unit residents with gamma globulin and feeding them the live hepatitis virus (obtained from the feces of … hepatitis patients)." At the same time a "control" group was "fed the live virus without the benefit of gamma globulin, to ascertain that the virus was actually 'live,' capable of transmitting the disease, and to measure the different responses" (Rothman and Rothman 1984: 16).

Consent forms that described the study in general terms were provided, but there is evidence that the parents' request to have their child admitted to the over-crowded institution would be denied if they did not consent. The extent to which consent was clearly explained or, in this manner, coerced, remains foggy. What was clear to Beecher, writing in 1966, was the study's violation of a resolution, extending the Nuremberg Code and adopted by the World Medical Association, that under no circumstances should a doctor be permitted to do anything to weaken the physical or mental resistance of a human being except in the interest of the patient. In no case was it acceptable to risk an injury to any person for the benefit of others.

Beecher's account of this intentional induction of hepatitis into institutionalized "mentally defective" children was included among 21 other projects of concern. As more information became available, the institution was identified as Willowbrook, the same over-crowded, squalid, poorly tended institution Senator Robert F. Kennedy had described in 1965 as bordering on a "snake pit."

In many ways, Willowbrook was a legacy of institutions for the "feebleminded" established in the heyday of the eugenics movement. The mandatory sterilization policies may have subsided, but residents were still seen as less worthy members of society and kept in conditions likened to dogs in a kennel. Beecher's account and Senator Robert Kennedy's characterization had only scratched the tip of a very much larger iceberg. The badly deteriorated, severely under-funded conditions and practices within the walls of Willowbrook remained out of the public's view.

In November of 1971, this lack of attention began to change. Local newspapers ran stories. A Willowbrook doctor had been organizing parents and staff to protest the abysmal conditions and mistreatment of children, an effort that got him fired. This same doctor approached a friend and local television reporter, Geraldo Rivera, asking that Rivera document the "horror" at Willowbrook. He wanted Rivera to see one section in particular where "there are sixty retarded kids, with only one attendant to take care of them. Most are naked and they lie in their own shit" (Rothman and Rothman 1984: 16). He had a key. He could get Rivera in.

Rivera's reporting of conditions in Willowbrook was aired in early January 1972. It captured national attention. As bad as the conditions at Willowbrook were, there was more to come. On July 25, 1972, some five months after a suit was filed on behalf of the residents at Willowbrook, another troubling story broke, this time in the *Washington Evening Star*. The headline read, "Syphilis Patients Died Untreated." The story was picked up nationwide and the next day the *New York Times* ran a parallel article: "Syphilis Victims in the U.S. Study Went Untreated for 40 Years." The lead sentence left little doubt:

> For 40 years the United States Public Health Service has conducted a study in which human beings with syphilis, who were induced to serve as guinea pigs, have gone without medical treatment for the disease and a few have died of its late effects, even though an effective therapy was eventually discovered." The study had begun in 1932, involving "about 600 black men, mostly poor and uneducated, from Tuskegee, Ala., an area that had the highest syphilis rate in the nation at the time.

If appalling institutional conditions and hepatitis research done on young retarded children on Staten Island and the radiation studies performed on cancer patients unable to secure alternative medical care in Cincinnati had awakened the conscience of some in Congress, it can rightly be said the account of the Tuskegee syphilis experiment scarred the Congressional soul. It is hard to imagine a more dramatic, inescapable example of the country's racist legacy than what took place in Macon County, Alabama over a 40-year period between 1932 and 1972.

Taken together, these three revelations of highly questionable medical research and practice left little doubt: some lives were deemed less worthy than others by the very physicians charged with their healing.[2] Some persons were less likely to be protected and their suffering was more likely to be tolerated. They could be used for the benefit of others—even if it meant the infliction of harm, suffering, and death.

Physicians and medical personnel involved in the Macon County syphilis study offered weak justifications that were difficult to sustain. Members of Congress reacted with shock. Senator William Proxmire, Democrat from Wisconsin, and a member of the Senate subcommittee that oversaw Public Health budgets, called the Tuskegee study "a moral and ethical nightmare" (quoted in Heller 1972). The assistant secretary of health and scientific affairs of the Department of Health, Education, and Welfare, when interviewed, reacted similarly. An official in the Venereal Disease Branch of the Center for Disease Control, where responsibility for the study resided in its final years, suggested, "a literal death sentence was passed on some of those people." "It is simply incredulous," he continued, "that such a thing could have ever happened. I honest to God don't understand it" (quoted in Jones 1981: 206–7).

It could no longer be easily argued, as Christiaan Bernard and others had done in Senator Mondale's 1968 hearings, that the common sense and professional judgment of physicians involved in research should be fully trusted. By November of 1972 a Science Policy Committee reported, "Never before have the issues [of medical research] been given such wide publicity or discussed so frankly as has been the case in recent months" (Science Policy Division, Congressional Research Service, Library of Congress 1972: 40). In a later thorough account, it was written, "More than any other experiment in American history, the Tuskegee study convinced legislators and bureaucrats alike that tough new regulations had to be adopted if human subjects were to be protected" (Jones 1981: 214).

---

2 As dramatic as these revelations were, there was still more. In July, 1973, *Relf v. Weinberger*, was filed in the District Court in the District of Columbia on behalf of two young, mentally retarded, black girls, ages 12 and 14, who had been involuntarily sterilized. During the hearings it was learned that an estimated 100,000 to 150,000 similarly situated cases had been sterilized annually under federally-funded programs. The effects of *Buck v. Bell* (1927) were alive and well. The District Court found such procedures to be "arbitrary and unreasonable" and ordered an end to the practice. As the case wound its way through the courts, federal regulations were changed to meet the new stricter standards for "informed consent" that were emerging. In 1977 *Relf* was remanded back to the District Court for dismissal, as the issue became moot. Parallel concerns were raised about the use of prisoners in medical research and the use of psychosurgery for behavior control. Psychosurgery for behavioral control had also become an issue depicted in the movie, *Clockwork Orange,* and Michael Chrichton's novel *The Terminal Man,* as well as a Februrary, 1973 article in *Ebony* magazine by Mason. See also, Veatch and Sollitto 1973: 1–3.

Senator Mondale's repeated calls for action would be further energized by one more recent account of ethically questionable science—the use of newly aborted fetuses in federally funded research. These came into sharp focus just months after the Supreme Court's landmark abortion decisions, in the *Washington Post* on April 10, 1973. The story prompted a phone call from Eunice Shriver, who was Executive Vice President of the Joseph P. Kennedy, Jr. Foundation, the prime benefactor of the Kennedy Institute. She was calling the Institute's director and friend, obstetrician, Dr. André Hellegers.

A visiting colleague at the Kennedy Institute, self-described as a recently appointed professor "in the fledging field of bioethics," was having lunch with Dr. Hellegers at the time. "As we were eating lunch, a waiter called him to the phone. After ten minutes, Dr. Hellegers returned, saying in his British-tinged Dutch accent, 'That was Eunice Shriver. She wanted to discuss what should be done to stop the fetal research that was reported in this morning's *Post*'" (Jonsen 1998: 94).

The *Washington Post* article, "Live-Fetus Research Debated," led with the sentence, "The possibility of using newly-delivered human fetuses—products of abortions—for medical research before they die is being strenuously debated by federal health officials." "Most scientists feel," the *Post* article continued, "that it is both moral and important to health progress to use some intact, living fetuses—fetuses too young and too small to live for any amount of time." Such tiny infants when delivered intact, often lived for an hour or so with beating heart after abortion. They could live longer without aid, primarily because their lungs were still unexpanded. But artificial aid, the article noted, "fresh blood and fresh oxygen—might keep them alive for three to four hours." A well-known genetics researcher was quoted in support of the research, "I do not think it's unethical. It is not possible to make this fetus into a child, therefore we can consider it as nothing more than a piece of tissue. It is the same principle as taking a beating heart from someone and making use of it in another person."

Others quoted in the article were not readily drawn to this analogy and instead turned to alternative comparisons, expressing deep empathy for the humanity of the fetus and drawing the boundaries of life quite differently. Using a not-yet-dead but soon-to-die fetus for medical research was more like experimenting on a person without their consent.

Prompted by the revelation of the Alabama syphilis study, the NIH had reopened the fetal research discussion. The parallels were readily apparent. Dr. Hellegers was quoted in opposition. "It appears that we want to make the chance for survival the reason for the experiment." When a colleague probed, "Isn't that the British approach?" Hellegers responded, "It was the German approach, 'If it is going to die, you might as well use it.'" Hellegers was concerned. The boundaries of protected life were important. They were being breached. "I include the live fetus inside the human race whether it is inside or outside the uterus." "Who are you to ask [for informed consent]," Hellegers asked, "the fetus that cannot give consent, or a mother who has already consented to the fetus' destruction?"

Where should the boundaries of protected life be drawn? How should the potential benefits of scientific research be balanced against competing values? Who should decide? These were gripping, profoundly important matters. They should not be left solely to the discretion of physicians and scientists doing the research. They were not to be dealt with behind closed doors, pressed this way or that by the politics of the moment. They should be fully aired in the light of day. Abiding principles, commanding public respect, were at stake.

Three days later a second article appeared in the *Washington Post* in which the National Institutes of Health gave assurances that it "does not now support" nor would it in the future support research on "live aborted human fetuses anyplace in the world." These assurances were made before an audience of some 200 Roman Catholic high school students. One of the young organizers of this gathering was 17-year-old Maria Shriver, daughter of Eunice Shriver, and later the First Lady of California.

The students were not altogether convinced. Referring to a federal advisory group who supported the continuation of "planned scientific studies" of the fetus under "carefully safeguarded" conditions, one student probed, "Why are they drawing up guidelines if they don't intend to use live fetuses?" It was a good question. It turned out the student's skepticism was justified. A third *Post* article, appearing two days later, reported that the NIH was in fact funding fetal research and that some researchers were doing their investigations by traveling to Finland and other countries where live fetuses and fetal tissue were more accessible.

Still, the NIH appeared to be tightening down, leading one advocate of continued fetal research to worry, "What I fear is that the new NIH action may make the situation so rigid that all research in this area may now be foreclosed." This would be a mistake. "Rather than it being immoral to do what we are trying to do, it is immoral—it is a terrible perversion of ethics—to throw these fetuses in the incinerator as is usually done, rather than to get some useful information." These same arguments would be heard some three decades later as molecular biology and associated technologies made it possible to engage in pluripotential stem cell research (see Guidelines for Human Embryonic Stem Cell Research 2005).

In 1973, however, attention was focused on mid-term fetuses. Should this still living but not yet viable tissue be used in research to advance life-enhancing knowledge? Or, were the fetuses fully protected members of the human family, infants not to be manipulated by researchers, even to advance the common good?

The civil rights implications of the Cincinnati, Willowbrook, and Tuskegee experiences, coupled with the abortion and right-to-life implications of the fetal research, created a powerful bipartisan coalition. Years later, Albert Jonsen, the "fledgling" bioethicist having lunch with Dr. Hellegers when he took the call from Eunice Shriver, had become the leading historian of the bioethics movement. He wrote how bipartisan support for the legislation was motivated by the two prominent cases of the moment. "The Tuskegee scandal cried out to liberals as a blatant violation of civil rights and an example of racism. The fetal research question, with its abortion implications, aroused conservatives in the pro-life camp" (Jonsen 1998: 98). The stage was set for what would be the first-ever legislation calling for a government body "to identify basic ethical principles."

The Search for Common Principles

This historic legislation (Public Law 93-348, the National Research Act) emerged when, in 1974, Walter Mondale's Senate colleague, Edward Kennedy, joined efforts with Representative Paul Rogers in the House. President Richard Nixon signed the bill into law in mid-July. Congress had established the National Commission for the Protection of Human Subjects of Biomedical and Behavioral Research. Eleven commission members were sworn in on December 3, 1974. The first order of business was to develop recommendations on fetal research as this was Congress's first priority and the legislation had placed a four-month deadline on this aspect of the report. In the end, the commissioners issued their report, closer to five months than four. Under specified conditions, fetal research could continue. One well-respected member of the commission submitted a reluctant but strongly worded dissent. He was not willing to consider the fetus less than human.

Once described as an "amiable, rumpled old bear" who "warmed the ground where he stood" (Coons 1978: 934), David Louisell, was a professor of law at the University of California, Berkeley. He was known for his kind demeanor and sharp wit, but also for his interest in the legal and moral implications of the biological revolution and strong opposition to the *Roe v. Wade* and *Doe v. Bolton* decisions released some two and a half years earlier (Louisell 1971, 1973; Louisell and Noonan 1970).

The commission had issued 16 recommendations, which dealt with therapeutic as well as nontherapeutic research directed toward the fetus and pregnant mother along with several provisions for the conduct of such research. Professor Louisell found two of these recommendations—#5 and #6—of particular concern. These allowed for "nontherapeutic research directed toward the fetus in anticipation of abortion" and "nontherapeutic research directed toward the fetus during the abortion procedure and the nontherapeutic research directed toward the nonviable fetus *ex utero*."

Professor Louisell concluded these recommendations were misguided, "insofar as they succumb to the error of sacrificing the interests of innocent human life to a postulated social need." He continued, "For me the lessons of history are too poignant, and those of this century too fresh, to ignore another violation of human integrity and autonomy by subjecting unconsenting human beings, whether or not viable, to harmful research even for laudable scientific purposes." Louisell's disagreement was not over the general ethical principles being applied by his colleagues. These he found to reflect "unquestioned morality." Rather, his objections were to where the boundaries of protected life were drawn and how the embedded dilemmas were balanced when the agreed upon general principles were applied to particular situations.

Recommendation #5 dealt with research on the fetus in anticipation of abortion. Given the Supreme Court's abortion decisions, this law professor knew he was on thin ice legally he asserted the personal autonomy and integrity of the non-viable fetus still in the womb. It did not matter. Abraham Lincoln's response to the *Dred Scott* decision, a ruling where persons of black African descent were declared non-citizens, came to mind. Louisell argued that like the *Dred Scott* decision, it was not necessary to extend the findings in *Roe* and *Doe* to other situations. Even if the Court had excluded the unborn from the full protective boundaries of personhood, we should resist extension of this idea to other contexts. Research on an unborn fetus, in anticipation of abortion, was an anathema. Professor Louisell could see "no legal principle which would justify, let alone require, passive submission to such a breach of our moral commitment."

Recommendation #6 was even more troubling. It spoke of the "nonviable fetus *ex utero.*" Up until that time, on both law and society, a nonviable fetus *ex utero* would have been seen simply "as an infant." In Louisell's judgment "all infants, however premature or inevitable their death, are within the norms governing human experimentation generally. We do not subject the aged dying to unconsented experimentation, nor should we the youthful dying."

Fetal research was only one section of the commission's report. In addition, the commission was charged with identifying more generally "the ethical principles which should underlie the conduct of biomedical and behavioral research with human subjects." Commission members convened to address this task in mid-February, 1976, some two years after being sworn in. They gathered at the Belmont House, in Elkridge Maryland, about a 45-minute drive outside the nation's capitol. The eventual report would take its name from this bucolic setting.

The Belmont Report and the Georgetown Principles

In 1977, after the 27th meeting of the commission, a group of commissioners, consultants, and staff convened in the San Francisco study of Albert Jonsen. The aim was to produce text that would be "succinct, easily comprehensible, and relevant to research practice" (Jonsen 2005). Three principles for medical research were settled upon—respect for persons (autonomy), beneficence, and justice. By design these principles and associated guidelines were general in nature and broad in scope. They had been gleaned from the specific problems addressed. On June 10, 1978, the commission at their 42nd gathering finally approved *The Belmont Report.*

A philosophy professor associated with the Kennedy Institute at Georgetown University, Tom Beauchamp, had been asked to join the staff and take responsibility for writing what was initially referred to simply as the "Belmont Paper." By his own account, he had no sense of the widespread and lasting impact this work would have. Instead he felt he "was the new-kid-on-the-block on the staff" and that he "was getting the dregs of the assignment. Because it was what nobody else wanted to do" (Oral History of the Belmont Report and the National Commission for the Protection of Human Subjects of Biomedical and Behavioral Research 2004: 6). While working in this capacity, Beauchamp began working with his colleague, Jim Childress, on what became their highly influential book, *Principles of Biomedical Ethics* (2009).

There was some disagreement on specifics, but in the end the *Belmont Report* and *Principles of Biomedical Ethics* were written simultaneously, the one influencing the other. By design, both aimed to encapsulate important elements of a "common morality," principles "shared by all morally decent persons," which were "woven into the fabric of morality in morally sensitive cultures" (Beauchamp 2003, 2005). Taken together, these overlapping works became highly influential benchmarks for bioethics. As attention increased, the framing importance of the principles enunciated, especially as developed by Beauchamp and Childress, would be referenced, and not always favorably, as the Georgetown Mantra.

When it came to the first principle, respect for persons or the idea of *autonomy*, most, even physicians directly involved in the recently revealed examples of disturbing medical research, would agree that individuals deserved respect as autonomous agents, and that persons with diminished capacities, such as children and the mentally handicapped, were entitled to protection. The second touchstone, *beneficence*, did not simply mean engaging in discretionary kindness or charity. Charity was a sought after virtue, but there was more. There was a strong obligation to secure the well-being of persons, to "do no harm," and to "maximize possible benefits and minimize possible harms." Finally, little disagreement would be found with the principle that *justice* should be advanced and protected. This seemed obvious. Given the injustices so evident in Cincinnati, Willowbrook, and Tuskegee, however, there was a need to underscore the obvious. There should be "fairness in distribution" of the benefits of medical research and selected categories of persons should not be asked to shoulder an unfair amount of the burden.

Though developed in the context of medical research, these principles were applicable to a wide range of related issues. They provided a "common coin of moral discourse." As a later observer, writing in the *Hastings Center Report* would put it, "The Babel of information formerly thought to be relevant to an ethical decision has been whittled down to a much more manageable level through the use of principles" (Evans 2000: 31). Still, questions and criticisms emerged (Clouser and Gert 1990). The enunciated principles of autonomy, beneficence, and justice failed as a straightforward guide to action. What did they mean in particular situations (Dubose, Hamel, and O'Connell 1994)? How did they help resolve the sometimes competing demands to alleviate intolerable suffering and to protect life?

Applying Moral Principles

Anchored in many ways with the logic, policies and practices of eugenics, disturbed by soul-searing Nazi atrocities, recognized in the reforms of a broad civil rights movement, and refined in encounters with disturbing medical experiments, a moral system evolved. As this shifting moral landscape was mapped, cases emerged in specific contexts and particular circumstances that tested the newly minted principles. Lacking an explicit ethical road map, specific decisions became works in progress. Checklists were developed to assist physicians and ethics committees (see Jonsen, Siegler, and Winslade 1998).

When the broad principles of the *Belmont Report* were applied within specific circumstances, competing conceptions of autonomy, beneficence, and justice emerged. Social movements were spawned to advance one point of view or another, issues were framed, power was exercised, and laws were crafted, appealed, and protested. These disagreements further refined the proposed principles. These refinements took place within debates over the legitimacy of abortion, the vagaries of neonatal care, the questions of assisted suicide, and the wisdom of laws calling for the full removal of autonomy and the execution of those convicted of capital crimes. Each of these topics is discussed in greater detail in subsequent volumes in this series.

DISCUSSION QUESTIONS

1. What do the Willowbrook, Tuskegee Syphilis, and Cincinnati radiation experiments have in common?
2. What other crystallizing events can you think of that have clarified thinking and motivated action?
3. Do you think that the government should regulate the research of physicians? Why or why not?
4. Do you think physicians should have ultimate say in how they interact with their patients?
5. What do you see as the pressing bioethical issues of our time? How are these different from or similar to those discussed in this chapter?

Bibliography

Books and Articles

Alexander, Leo. 1949. "Medical Science Under Dictatorship." *The New England Journal of Medicine* *241*(2): 39–47.

Alexander, Shana. 1962. "They Decide Who Lives, Who Dies: Medical Miracle and a Moral Burden of a Small Committee." *Life* (November 9): 103–28.

Allen, Garland E. 1986. "The Eugenics Record Office at Cold Spring Harbor, 1910–1940: An Essay in Institutional History." *Osiris 2*: 225–64.

Alschuler, Albert W. 2000. *Law Without Values: The Life, Work, and Legacy of Justice Holmes*. Chicago: University of Chicago Press.

Atlanta Constitution. 1997. (July 26): 1.A.

Auerbach, Stuart. 1971. "Faculty Study Hits Whole-Body Radiation Plan" A3. University Archives, University of Cinncinatti.

Barrett, Deborah, and Charles Kurzman. 2004. "Globalizing Social Movement Theory: The Case of Eugenics." *Theory and Society 33*: 487–527.

Beauchamp, Tom. 2003. "The Origins, Goals, and Core Commitments of *The Belmont Report and Principles of Biomedical Ethics*." Pp. 17–46 in *The Story of Bioethics: From Seminal Works to Contemporary Explorations*, eds. Jennifer K. Walter and Eran P. Klein. Washington D.C.: Georgetown University Press:

———. 2005. "The Origins and Evolution of the *Belmont Report*." Pp. 12–25 in *Belmont Revisited: Ethical Principles for Research with Human Subjects*, eds. James F. Childress, Eric M. Meslin, and Harold T. Shapiro. Washington D.C.: Georgetown University Press.

Beauchamp, Tom L., and James F. Childress. 2001. *Principles of Biomedical Ethics,* 5th ed. New York: Oxford University Press.

———. 2009. *Principles of Biomedical Ethics,* 6th ed. New York: Oxford University Press.

Beecher, Henry K. 1959. "Experimentation in Man," *Journal of the American Medical Association 169*: 461–78.

———. 1968. "Medical Research and the Individual." P. 16 in *Life or Death: Ethics and Options*, ed. Daniel Labby. Seattle: University of Washington Press.

———. 1999. "Ethics and Clinical Research." Pp. 79–90 in *Bioethics: An Anthology*, eds. Helga Kuhse and Peter Singer. New York: Wiley-Blackwell.

Beicken, Julie. 2009. *Eugenics: An Elite Social Movement*. Masters Thesis, University of Texas, Austin.

Bishop, E., and W. F. Nelms. 1930. "A Simple Method of Tubal Sterilization." *New York State Journal of Medicine 30*: 214–16.

Black, Edwin. 2003. *War Against the Weak: Eugenics and America's Campaign to Create a Master Race*. New York: Four Walls Eight Windows.

Blagg, C. R. 1998. "Development of Ethical Concepts in Dialysis: Seattle in the 1960s." *Nephrology 4*: 236.

Bradley, Omar. 1977. *The Collected Writings of General Omar N. Bradley*, Vol. 1: Speeches 1945–1949. Washington, D.C.: U.S. Government Printing Office.

Callahan, Daniel. 1973. "Bioethics as a Discipline." *The Hastings Center Studies 1*: 66–73.

Carmody, James. 1970. *Ethical Issues in Health Services: A Report and Annotated Bibliography*. Washington D.C.: National Center for Health Services Research and Development.

Chalmers, David. 1987. *Hooded Americanism*, 3rd ed. Durham: Duke University Press.

Clouser, K. Danner, and Bernard Gert. 1990. "A Critique of Principlism." *The Journal of Medicine and Philosophy 15*: 219–36.

Coons, John E. 1978. "David W. Louisell, In Memoriam." *California Law Review 66*: 934.

Crichton, Michael. 2009. *A Terminal Man*. New York: Harper.

Dartmouth Alumni Magazine. 1960. *53*(2): 7–8.

Darwin, Charles. 1876. *The Autobiography of Charles Darwin*, ed. by N. Barlow. London: Collins.

Davenport, Charles B. 1912. *Eugenics Record Office Bulletin No. 6, The Trait Book*. Cold Spring Harbor, NY.

Dubose, Edwin R., Ronald P. Hamel, and Laurence J. O'Connell, eds. 1994. *A Matter of Principles? Ferment in U.S. Bioethics*. Valley Forge, PA: The Trinity Press International.

Ekland-Olson, Sheldon. 2012. *Who Lives, Who Dies, Who Decides?* New York: Routledge.

Estabrook, Arthur H. 1916. *The Jukes in 1915*. Washington, DC: Carnegie Institute of Washington.

"Eugenical Sterilization in Germany." 1933. *Eugenical News 18*: 89–94.

Eugenics Record Office. 1911. *Bulletin No. 1 Heredity of Feeble-Mindedness*. Cold Spring Harbor, NY.

———. 1914. *Bulletin No. 10A: Report to the Committee to Study and to Report on the Best Practical Means of Cutting Off the Defective Germ Plasm in the American Population: The Scope of the Committee's Work,* Cold Spring Harbor, NY.

———. 1914. Bulletin No. 10B: Report to the Committee to Study and to Report on the Best Practical Means of Cutting Off the Defective Germ Plasm in the American Population: The Legal, Legislative and Administrative Aspects of Sterilization. Cold Spring Harbor, NY.

Evans, John H. 2000. "A Sociological Account of the Growth of Principlism." *Hastings Center Report 3*: 31–38.

Farley, Margaret. 2002. Foreword to *The Patient as Person: Explorations in Medical Ethics* (2nd ed.), ed. Paul Ramsey. New Haven: Yale University Press: xi–xiiv

Fletcher, Joseph. 1954. *Morals and Medicine*. Princeton: Princeton University Press.

Foot, Philippa. 1967. "The Problem of Abortion and the Doctrine of the Double Effect." *Oxford Review 5*: 5–15.

Fuller, Lon. 1949. "The Case of the Speluncean Explorers." *Harvard Law Review 62*: 616–45.

Galton, Francis. 1869. *Hereditary Genius*. New York: MacMillan and Company.

———. 1883. *Inquiries into Human Faculty and its Development.* New York: J.M. Dent & Co. London and E.P. Dutton & Co.

———. 1901. "The Possible Improvement of the Human Breed Under the Existing Conditions of Law and Sentiment," The Second Huxley Lecture of the Anthropological Institute, delivered on October 29.

———. 1904. "Eugenics: Its Definition, Scope, and Aims." *The American Journal of Sociology 10*: 1–27.

———. 1908. *Memories of My Life.* London: Methuen.

Gerdtz, John. 2006. "Disability and Euthanasia: The Case of Helen Keller and the Bollinger Baby" (paper presented at the sixteenth University Faculty for Life Conference).

Goddard, Henry Herbert. 1912. *The Kallikak Family: A Study in the Heredity of Feeble-Mindedness.* New York: The Macmillian Company.

Gosney, E. S., and Paul Popenoe. 1929. *Sterilization for Human Betterment.* New York: The Macmillian Company.

Granovetter, Mark. 1983. "The Strength of Weak Ties: A Network Theory Revisited." *Sociological Theory 1*: 201–33.

Grant, Madison. 1916. *The Passing of the Great Race.* New York: Charles Scribner's Sons.

Guidelines for Human Embryonic Stem Cell Research. 2005. Washington D.C. National Academies Press.

Gustafson, James. 1968. "Review of *Life or Death: Ethics and Options.*" *Commonweal 89*: 27–30.

Hall, Jacquelyn H,, and David D. Swenson. 1968. *Psychological and Social Aspects of Human Tissue Transplantation: Annotated Bibliography.* Washington, D.C.: U.S. Department of Health, Education, and Welfare.

Harvey, C. P. 1967. "Ethics in Medical Progress: A Ciba Foundation Symposium." *The Modern Law Review 30*: 591–93.

Heller, Jean. 1972. "Syphilis Victims in the U.S. Study Went Untreated for 40 Years." *The New York Times* (July 26).

Hume, D. M., et al. 1963. "Renal Homotransplantation in Man in Modified Recipients." *Annals of Surgery 158*: 608–44

Huxley, Aldous. 1993. *Brave New World.* New York: Harper Collins.

Jones, James H. 1981. *Bad Blood: The Tuskegee Syphilis Experiment.* New York: The Free Press.

Jonsen, Albert R. 1990. *The New Medicine & The Old Ethics.* Cambridge, MA.: Harvard University Press.

———. 1993. "The Birth of Bioethics." *Special Supplement, Hastings Center Report 23*(6): S1, S16.

———. 1998. *The Birth of Bioethics.* New York: Oxford University Press.

———. 2002. "The Structure of an Ethical Revolution: Paul Ramsey, the Beecher Lectures, and the Birth of Bioethics." Pp. xvi–xxvii in *The Patient as Person: Explorations in Medical Ethics, 2nd ed.,* ed. Paul Ramsey. New Haven: Yale University Press.

———. 2005. "On the Origins and Future of the Belmont Report." Pp. 3–11 in *Belmont Revisited: Ethical Principles for Research with Human Subjects,* ed. James F. Childress, Eric M. Meslin, and Harold T. Shapiro. Washington, D.C.: Georgetown University Press.

Jonsen, Albert R., Mark Siegler, and William Winslade. 1998. *Clinical Ethics*, 4th ed. New York: McGraw Hill Companies.

Jordan, David Starr. 1907. *The Human Harvest: A Study of the Decay of Races Through the Survival of the Unfit*. Cambridge: American Unitarian Association.

Kass, Leon R. 2002. *Life, Liberty and the Defense of Dignity: The Challenge of Bioethics*. San Francisco: Encounter Books.

Keller, Helen. 1915. "Physicians' Juries for Defective Babies." *The New Republic 18* (December): 173–74.

Kennedy, Foster. 1942. "The Problem of Social Control of the Congenitally Defective: Education, Sterilization, Euthanasia." *American Journal of Psychiatry 99*: 13–16.

Kevles, Daniel. 1985. *In the Name of Eugenics*. New York: Knopf.

Kimmelman, Barbara A. 1983. "The American Breeders' Association: Genetics and Eugenics in an Agricultural Context, 1903–13." *Social Studies of Science 13*: 163–204.

Kühl, Stefan. 1994. *The Nazi Connection: Eugenics, American Racism, and German National Socialism*. New York: Oxford University Press.

Labby, Daniel, ed. 1966. *Life or Death: Ethics and Options*. Seattle: University of Washington Press.

Lankester, Sir Edwin Ray. 1880. *Degeneration, A Chapter in Darwinism*. London: Macmillian.

Laughlin, Harry. 1922. *Eugenical Sterilization in the United States*. Chicago: Psychopathic Laboratory of the Municipal Court of Chicago.

Lifton, Robert Jay. 1986. *The Nazi Doctors: Medical Killing and the Psychology of Genocide*. New York: Basic Books.

Little, Jr., Richard N. 1972. "Experimentation with Human Subjects: Legal and Moral Considerations Regarding Radiation Treatment of Cancer at the University of Cincinnati College of Medicine." *Atomic Energy Law Journal 13*: 305–30.

Lombardo, Paul A. 1985. "Three Generations, No Imbeciles: New Light on *Buck v. Bell*." *New York University Law Review 60*: 30–62.

Louisell, David. 1971. "Biology, Law and Reason: Man as Self-Creator." *American Journal of Jurisprudence* 1–16.

———. 1973. "Euthanasia and Banthasia: On Dying and Killing." *Catholic University Law Review 22*: 723, 737.

Louisell, David, and John T. Noonan. 1970. "Constitutional Balance." Pp. 113–27 in *The Morality of Abortion: Legal and Historical Perspectives*, John T. Noonan, ed. Cambridge: Harvard University Press.

Mason, B. J. 1973. "Brain Surgery to Control Behavior." *Ebony*: 63–72.

McCoy, Alfred W. 2006. *A Question of Torture: CIA Interrogation, From the Cold War to the War on Terror*. New York: Henry Holt.

McElhinney, Thomas K., and Edmund D. Pellegrino. 2001. "The Institute of Human Values in Medicine: Its Role and Influence in the Conception and Evolution of Bioethics." *Theoretical Medicine 22*: 291–317.

Mead, Margaret. 1957. "Toward More Vivid Utopias." *Science 126*: 957–61.

Memorandum issued by the Research Grants Division of United States Public Health Services on Feb. 8, 1966, Statement of Policy.

Murray, J. E., et al. 1962. "Kidney Transplantation in Modified Recipients." *Annals of Surgery 156*: 337–55.

———. 1963. "Prolonged Survival of Human Kidney Homografts by Immunosuppressive Drug Therapy." *New England Journal of Medicine 268*: 1315–23.

Ochsner, Albert J. 1899. "Surgical Treatment of Habitual Criminals." *Journal of the American Medical Association 53*: 867–68.

Ogburn, William. 1964. *On Culture and Social Change,* ed. Otis Dudley Duncan. Chicago: The University of Chicago Press.

Oral History of the Belmont Report and the National Commission for the Protection of Human Subjects of Biomedical and Behavioral Research. 2004. Retrieved March 2009 (http://www.hhs.gov/ohrp/archive/belmontArchive.html).

Pappworth, M. H. 1962. "Human Guinea Pigs: A Warning." *The Twentieth Century*: 66–75.

Paul, Diane B. 1995. *Controlling Human Heredity – 1865 to the Present.* Atlantic Highlands, NJ: Humanities Press.

Pernick, Martin S. 1996).*The Black Stork: Eugenics and the Death of "Defective" Babies in American Medicine and Motion Pictures since 1915.* New York: Oxford University Press.

Pius XI. 1939. "On Christian Marriage." Pp. 96–97 in *Five Great Encyclicals.* New York: Paulist Press.

Popenoe, Paul, and Roswell Johnson. 1918. *Applied Eugenics.* New York: The Macmillan Company.

Potter, Van Rensselaer. 1971. *Bioethics Bridge to the Future.* New York: Prentice Hall.

Reich, Warren Thomas. 1994. "The Word 'Bioethics': Its Birth and the Legacies of Those Who Shaped Its Meaning." *Kennedy Institute of Ethics Journal 4*: 319–35

———. 1995. "The Word 'Bioethics': The Struggle over Its Earliest Meanings." *Kennedy Institute of Ethics Journal 5*: 19–34.

Reilly, Philip R. 1987. "Involuntary Sterilization in the United States: A Surgical Solution." *The Quarterly Review of Biology 62*: 153–70.

———. 1991. *The Surgical Solution: A History of Involuntary Sterilization in the United States.* Baltimore: Johns Hopkins University Press.

"The Rockefeller Foundation and the Kaiser Wilhelm Institute." 1936. *Science 84*: 526–27.

Rogers, Daniel. 1982. "In Search of Progressivism." *Reviews in American History 10*: 113–32.

Rothman, David J. 1991. *Strangers at the Bedside: A History of How Law and Bioethics Transformed Medical Decision Making.* New York: Basic Books.

Rothman, David J., and Sheila M. Rothman. 1984. *The Willowbrook Wars.* New York: Harper and Row.

The Sanctity of Life. 1966. Symposium (March 11–12). Reed College, Portland, Oregon.

Sanders, David, and Jesse Dukeminier, Jr. 1968. "Medical Advance and Legal Lag: Hemodialysis and Kidney Transplantation." *UCLA Law Review 15*: 357–413.

Science Policy Division, Congressional Research Service, Library of Congress. 1972. "Genetic Engineering, Evolution of a Technological Issue." Report to the Subcommittee on Science, Research and Development, House Committee on Science and Astronautics (November, 8): 40.

Scribner, Belding H. 1964. "Ethical Problems of Using Artificial Organs to Sustain Human Life." *Transactions-American Society for Artificial Internal Organs 10*: 209–12.

Sharp, Harry C. 1902. "The Severing of the Vasa Differentia and its Relation to the Neuropsychiatric Constitution." *New York Medical Journal 46*: 411–14.

———. 1907. Vasectomy as a Means of Preventing Procreation of Defectives." *Journal of American Medical Association 51*: 1897–1902.

Snow, David A., Louis, A. Zurcher, and Sheldon Ekland-Olson. 1980. "Social Networks and Social Movements: A Micro-Structural Approach to Differential Recruitment." *American Sociological Review 45*: 789.

Starzl, T. E., T. L. Marchioro, and W. R. Waddell. 1963. "The Reversal of Rejection in Human Renal Homografts with Subsequent Development of Homograft Tolerance." *Surgery, Gynecology, and Obstetrics 117*: 385–95

Stephens, Jerome. 1973. "Political, Social, and Scientific Aspects of Medical Research on Humans." *Politics and Society 3*: 409–27.

Stephens, Martha. 2002. *The Treatment: The Story of Those Who Died in the Cincinnati Radiation Tests.* Durham: Duke University Press.

Stern, Alexandra Minna. 2005. *Eugenic Nation: Faults & Frontiers of Better Breeding in Modern America.* Berkeley: University of California Press.

———. 2007. "'We Cannot Make a Silk Purse Out of a Sow's Ear': Eugenics in the Hoosier Heartland." *Indiana Magazine of History 103*: 3–38.

Stevens, M. L. Tina. 2000. *Bioethics in America: Origins and Cultural Politics.* Baltimore: Johns Hopkins University Press.

Thomson, Judith Jarvis. 1971. "A Defense of Abortion." *Philosophy & Public Affairs 1*: 47–66.

———. 1976. "Killing, Letting Die, and the Trolley Problem." *The Monist 59*: 204–17.

Tolnay, Stewart E., and E. M. Beck. 1995 *A Festival of Violence: An Analysis of Southern Lynchings, 1882–1930.* Urbana and Chicago: University of Illinois Press.

Tooley, Michael. 1972. "Abortion and Infanticide." *Philosophy and Public Affairs 2*: 37–65.

Veatch, Robert M., and Sharmon Sollitto. 1973. "Human Experimentation: The Ethical Questions Persist." *The Hastings Center Report 3*: 1–3.

Wechsler, Herbert. 1952. "The Challenge of a Model Penal Code." *Harvard Law Review 65*: 1098–1127.

Weeks, Genevieve C. 1976. *Oscar Carleton McCulloch 1843–1891: Teacher and Practitioner of Applied Christianity.* Indianapolis: Indianapolis Historical Society.

Weingart, Peter. 1989. "German Eugenics Between Science and Politics." *Osiris*, 2nd Series 5: 260–82.

Welsome, Eileen. 1999. *The Plutonium Files: America's Secret Medical Experiments in the Cold War.* New York: The Dial Press, Random House.

Wolfensberger, Wolf. 1975. *The Origin and Nature of Our Institutional Models.* Syracuse: Human Policy Press.

Woodard, P. S., ed. 2001. *The Doctrine of Double Effect: Philosophers Debate a Controversial Moral Principle.* Notre Dame: University of Notre Dame Press.

Woodruff, M .F. et al. 1963. "Homotransplantation of Kidney in Patients Treated by Preoperative Local Radiation and Postoperative Administration of an Antimetabolite." *Lancet 2*: 675–82.

Woods, Frederick Adams. 1918. "The Passing of the Great Race." *Science* (October 25): 419–20.

Conference Presentations and Speeches

Gerdtz, John. 2006. "Disability and Euthanasia: The Case of Helen Keller and the Bollinger Baby." Presented at the sixteenth University Faculty for Life Conference.

Huxley, Aldous. (October 29, 1901) "The Possible Improvement of the Human Breed Under the Existing Conditions of Law and Sentiment." Presented at the Second Huxley Lecture of the Anthropological Institute.

Irving, Dianne N. 2000. "What is Bioethics?" Presented at the American Bioethics Advisory Commission, Washington, D.C.

Court Cases

Buck v. Bell 274 U.S. 200 (1927).

Doe v. Bolton, 410 U.S. 179 (1973).

Haynes v. Lapeer Cir. Judge, 201 Mich. 138, 144-45, 166 N.W.938, 940-41 (1918).

Loving v. Virginia, 388 U.S. 1 (1967).

Osborne v. Thomson, 103, Misc. 23, 33-36, 169 N.Y.S. 638,643-45, aff'd; 185 App. Div. 902, 171 N.Y.S. 1094 (1918).

Relf v. Weinberger, 372 F. Supp. 1196 - Dist. Court, 1974.

Roe v. Wade, 410 U.S. 113 (1973).

Smith v. Board of Examiners of Feeble-Minded. 88 A. 963 (1913).

Films

The Lynchburg Story: Eugenic Sterilization in America. 1994. Stephen Trombley, Director; Bruce Eadie, Producer. Worldview Pictures Production.

Unforgotten: Twenty-Five Years After Willowbrook. 2010. Jack Fisher, Director (City Lights Pictures).

Websites

"Elmira." (N.D.). Accessed online at http://www.correctionhistory.org/html/chronicl/docs2day/elmira.html

"Nuremberg Code." (N.D.). Accessed online at http://www.jewishvirtuallibrary.org/jsource/Holocaust/Nuremberg_Code.html lhttp://www.hhs.gov/ohrp/archive/belmontArchive.html

Glossary/Index

A

ABA (American Breeders' Association) 8, 13–14

abortion 41, 42, 46, 55, 56–57, 58, 60

"Act for the Prevention of Idiocy" 17–18

Admissions Advisory Committee 37

    AES (American Eugenics Society) 8, 22

Alexander, Leo 35, 36, 43, 47

Alexander, Shana 37, 38

American Genetics Association 8, 14

American Society for Artificial Internal Organs 36

autonomy: a person's ability to make his/her own decision. In relation to medicine and ethics, the concept refers to physicians or researchers providing patients or subjects with the most accurate information so that they can make the best decisions for themselves and resist coercion. In addition to beneficence and justice, one of the three principles of bioethics written in *The Belmont Report*. 3, 18, 25, 26, 33, 57, 58, 59, 60

B

Barr, M. W. 12

Beauchamp, Tom 58, 59

Beecher, Henry K. 42–44, 45, 47, 52, 53

Bell, Alexander Graham 10

Bell, James H.

    See Buck v. Bell

Belmont Report, The 44, 58–60

beneficence: more than engaging in discretionary kindness or charity, beneficence refers to the obligation to maximize benefits and minimize harms. In addition to autonomy and justice, beneficence was one of the three principles to guide bioethics written in *The Belmont Report*. 18, 58, 59, 60

Bennis, Warren 52

Bernard, Christiaan 44, 45, 54
Better Baby Contests 22
Binet, Alfred 14
bioethics: the discipline that explores issues of morality and ethics in relation to science, medicine, and technology 18, 37, 41–42, 46, 47, 48, 49, 50, 55, 56, 59
Bioethics (Potter) 48
Birth of a Nation, The (Dixon) 21
Black Stork, The (film) 21
Blood of a Nation, The (Jordan) 13
Boas, Franz 16, 27
Bradley, Omar 34
Brain Death Committee 45
Brave New World (Huxley) 36
Buck Carrie 16, 28–30, 33
Buck v. Bell 1–2, 24, 26, 29–30, 31, 32, 51, 54
Burbank, Luther 10

C
Cahn, Edmond 40–41
Callahan, Daniel 49
Carnegie Institute of Washington 10
Childress, Jim 59
Cincinnati Radiation Study 50–51, 56, 59, 60
Civil Rights Act of 20, 1871
Clansmen, The (Dixon) 21
Crampton, Harry 22
crystallizing event: important events that clarify issues and motivate action. Frequently occurrences that change the course of history and call for rethinking of moral standards and ethical understandings of how society should be structured and its members should treat one another. Crystallizing events often result in amending or creating legislation and policy and contribute to the evolution of moral systems. 1, 2, 36, 37, 48, 50–60
cultural lag: the idea that when science and technology advance rapidly, it takes longer for culture to catch up. Thus there is a disconnect between what science and technology enables us to do and the moral systems we use to assess these decisions. 35–36, 45, 47

D
Darvall, Denise Ann 44–45
Darwin, Charles 1, 4, 5, 8
Davenport, Charles Benedict 8–10, 14, 16, 25

Declaration of Helsinki 43

degenerates: as used in the eugenics movement, members of society that were considered unfit and undesirable to the nation. Included groups such as the blind, deaf, mute, paupers, epileptic, feebleminded, prostitutes, alcoholics, etc. These groups were the targets of eugenics efforts. 4, 17, 18

DeJarnette, Joseph 28

Dixon, Thomas 21

Doctrine of Double Effect: Doctrine of the Catholic Church generally attributed to Thomas Aquinas. Intending good, knowing harm will result is morally acceptable. 41, 47, 74

Doe v. Bolton 25, 57

Dred Scott v. Sandford 58

Dugdale, Richard 11, 14

E

ERO (Eugenics Record Office) 1, 8–10, 13, 16, 31, 35

Estabrook, Arthur 15–16, 26, 28

Eugenics Committee of the American Breeders' Association 9, 10

Eugenics Research Association 25

euthanasia: assisting in the death of someone who is suffering. In eugenic terms, that suffering could mean they were not a fit member of society. 22, 35, 41

F

Fischer, Eugen 32

Fitter Family Contests 22

Foot-Notes to Evolution (McCulloch) 13

Foot, Philippa 41

Fuller, Lon 40

G

Galton, Francis 5–7, 8, 11

Galton Society, The 8

Garrison, Judge 23, 31, 33

Georgetown Principles of Bioethics 18, 58–59

Gilligan, John 52

Goddard, Henry 14–15, 23, 26

Gosney, E. S. 22, 23, 31

Grant, Madison 16, 20, 22, 25

Gustafson, James 46

H

Haiseldon, Harry 21

Hanley, J. Frank 18, 19

Harriman, Edward Henry 9

Harriman Foundation 9, 10

Harriman, Mary 9

Hastings Center Report, The 49, 50, 59

Hastings Center, The 49, 50

Heidelberg University 17

Hellegers, André 55, 56

hemodialysis: the process of flushing out the kidneys by machine for persons with advanced renal disease, when the kidneys are no longer capable of doing it themselves 39, 40, 41, 42

Hitler, Adolf 2, 16, 17, 31, 32

Holmes, Oliver Wendell 1–2, 26, 29–30, 31, 51

Human Betterment Foundation 8, 22–23, 30, 31, 32

Hurty, John 19

Huxley, Aldous 36

I

idiot: one of the categories of intelligence, just below imbecile, created by psychologist Henry Goddard. Idiot refers to a person with inadequate mental capacity. 14, 23

imbecile: one of the categories of intelligence, just below moron, created by psychologist Henry Goddard. Imbecile is a category for someone with inadequate mental capacity. 2, 12, 14, 23, 29

Indianapolis Congregational Church 10

indiscriminate benevolence 7

J

JAMA (Journal of the American Medical Association) 43

JFA (Junior Faculty Association) report 51–52

Jim Crow Laws 20, 22

Jonsen, Albert 41, 56, 58

Jordan, David Starr 10, 13, 14, 16, 18, 19, 22

Jukes family study 11, 14, 15

justice: in addition to autonomy and beneficence, one of the three principles to guide bioethics written in *The Belmont Report*. In this context, justice refers to the fair and equitable distribution of treatment and the benefits of medical research, and that additionally, no particular groups should be disproportionately tested. 18, 58, 59, 60

Moral Decision, The (Cahn) 40

moron: one of the categories of intelligence, just above imbecile in intelligence, created by psychologist Henry Goddard 14, 23, 27

Muller, Hermann Joseph 27

Murray, Joseph 44, 45

N

National Commission for the Protection of Human Subjects of Biomedical and Behavioral Research 44, 57, 59

Nazism 2, 3, 16, 17, 35

negative eugenics: a movement in the late nineteenth and early twentieth century to rid society of undesirable characteristics by reducing reproduction of groups of persons considered unfit and quelling immigration from undesirable points of origin 7, 16

New England Journal of Medicine 35, 44, 52

NIH (National Institutes of Health) 55, 56

Nixon, Richard 57

Nuremberg Code 35, 43, 47, 52

Nuremberg Trials 2, 18

O

Olson, Harry 23, 25, 26, 28

Origin of the Species (Darwin) 4

Osborne, Henry Fairfield 22

P

Passing of the Great Race, The (Grant) 16, 20–21, 22

Patient as Person, The (Ramsey) 47

Pearson, Karl 5, 6, 8

Pennypacker, Samuel 18, 24, 31, 33, 49

Pomery method, tubal ligation 30

Popenoe, Paul 14, 22, 23, 31

positive eugenics: encouraging better marriages and taking other measures for the purpose of producing non-degenerate offspring 7

Potter, Van Rensselaer 48, 49

Priddy, Albert 26–29, 33

Principles of Biomedical Ethics (Beauchamp and Childress) 59

Proxmire, William 54

R

Race Betterment Foundation 8, 22

Racial Integrity Act 25, 26
Ramsey, Paul 46, 47, 50
Reed College 42, 43
Relf v. Weinberger 54
Rivera, Geraldo 53
Rockefeller Foundation 32, 35
Roe v. Wade 25, 57, 58
Roger, Paul 57
Rüdin, Ernst 32

S
Saenger, Eugene 50
salpingectomy 23, 26
Sanctity of Life conference 42–43
Scribner, Belding 36, 37
Seattle Artificial Kidney Center 37
SESE (Station for the Experimental Study of Evolution) 8, 9
Sharp, Harry 18, 19
Shriver, Eunice 55, 56
Shriver, Maria 56
Simon-Binet Scale: a scale developed by Theodore Simon and Alfred Binet to measure people's mental capacity and intelligence. This scale ultimately became what we know as the IQ (intelligence quotient) test. 14
Simon, Theodore 14
Smith, Alice 23, 24
social worth: a person's assessed value to society, nation, and the community in which they live 24, 33, 34, 37–38, 39, 40, 41, 51
Society of Health and Human Values 49
Standing Committee on Human Studies 44
Stephens, Martha 51, 52
Sterilization Act 25–26, 29
Sterilization for Human Betterment (Gosney and Popenoe) 23, 31
sterilization, mandatory 11, 16, 17–22, 23–25, 30–32, 35, 49, 51, 53
Strode, Aubrey 26, 28, 29, 33

T
Terman, Lewis 14
"The Jukes:" A Study in Crime, Pauperism, Disease and Heredity 11
Trait Book, The (Davenport) 14
Tribe of Ishmael, The: A Study of Social Degradation (McCulloch) 11–12, 13

trolley problem: a philosophical ethical dilemma designed in part to reveal the Doctrine of Double Effect. Generally, in The Trolley Problem, people are forced to choose how a trolley goes down a track. They are given two options. One results in the death of one person; the other results in the death of some multiple of persons. In different situations, the characteristics of the persons are varied. People must place value on life, weighing social worth in deciding whether to spare one life or others. 41

U

unintended consequences: results that may occur without being desired. For example, an unintended consequence of the development of the hemodialysis machine was having to come up with criteria for hierarchically ranking people based on who should have access to the treatment. 41

V

W

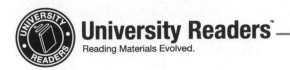
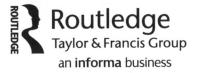